ABC OF
CLINICAL HAEMATOLOGY

Second Edition

ABC OF
CLINICAL HAEMATOLOGY

Second Edition

Edited by

DREW PROVAN

Senior Lecturer, Department of Haematology, Bart's and the London,
Queen Mary's School of Medicine and Dentistry, London

© BMJ Books 2003
BMJ Books is an imprint of the BMJ Publishing Group

First published in 1998
Second edition 2003

by BMJ Books, BMA House, Tavistock Square,
London WC1H 9JR

www.bmjbooks.com

British Library Cataloguing in Publication Data
A catalogue record for this book is available from the British Library

ISBN 0 7279 16769

Typeset by Newgen Imaging Systems (P) Ltd., Chennai, India
Printed and bound in Spain by GraphyCems, Navarra

Cover image: False colour SEM of blood with myeloid leukaemia.
Robert Becker/Custom Medical Stock Photo/Science Photo Library.

Contents

Contributors

Andrew Duncombe
Consultant Haematologist, Southampton University Hospitals NHS Trust, Southampton

Tyrrell G J R Evans
Senior Lecturer, Department of General Practice and Primary Care, King's College School of Medicine and Dentistry, London

T Everington
Specialist Registrar, Department of Haematology, University College London Hospitals NHS Trust, London

Adele K Fielding
Senior Associate Consultant and Assistant Professor in Medicine, Molecular Medicine Program and Division of Hematology, Mayo Clinic, Rochester, MN, USA

John Goldman
Professor of Haematology, Imperial College School of Medicine, Hammersmith Hospital, London

A H Goldstone
Consultant Haematologist, Department of Haematology, University College London Hospitals NHS Trust, London

Anthony R Green
Professor of Haemato-Oncology, Department of Haematology, Cambridge Institute for Medical Research, Cambridge

K K Hampton
Senior Lecturer in Haematology, Royal Hallamshire Hospital, Sheffield

Victor Hoffbrand
Emeritus Professor of Haematology and Honorary Consultant Haematologist, Royal Free Hospital Hampstead NHS Trust and School of Medicine, London

R J Liesner
Consultant Haematologist, Department of Haematology and Oncology, Great Ormond Street Hospital for Children NHS Trust, London, and Department of Haematology, University College London Hospitals NHS Trust, London

S J Machin
Professor of Haematology, Department of Haematology, University College London Hospitals NHS Trust, London

G M Mead
Consultant in Medical Oncology, Wessex Medical Oncology Unit, Southampton University Hospitals NHS Trust, Southampton

Adrian C Newland
Professor of Haematology, Department of Haematology, Bart's and the London, Queen Mary's School of Medicine and Dentistry, London

David G Oscier
Consultant Haematologist, Department of Haematology and Oncology, Royal Bournemouth Hospital, Bournemouth, and Honorary Senior Lecturer, University of Southampton

F E Preston
Professor of Haematology, Royal Hallamshire Hospital, Sheffield

Drew Provan
Senior Lecturer, Department of Haematology, Bart's and the London, Queen Mary's School of Medicine and Dentistry, London

Stephen J Russell
Director, Molecular Medicine Program, Mayo Foundation, Rochester, MN, USA

Charles R J Singer
Consultant Haematologist, Royal United Hospital, Bath

George S Vassiliou
Leukaemia Research Fund Clinical Research Fellow/Honorary Specialist Registrar, Department of Haematology, Cambridge Institute for Medical Research, Cambridge

Sir David J Weatherall
Regius Professor of Medicine Emeritus, Weatherall Institute of Molecular Medicine, University of Oxford, John Radcliffe Hospital, Oxford

Preface

As with most medical specialties, haematology has seen major changes since this book was first published in 1998. We now have greater understanding of the molecular biology of many diseases, both malignant and non-malignant. This new knowledge has helped us to develop more sensitive assays for many conditions, and has been taken into the clinic, with the engineering of new drugs, such as STI571 used in the treatment of chronic myeloid leukaemia, amongst others.

As with the first edition, the intention has been to encompass all aspects of haematology but with perhaps a greater emphasis on basic science than previously. Readers will note that the writing team is almost identical to that for the first edition, which provides continuity of style.

I would like to express my gratitude to all my haematology colleagues for updating their sections and bringing the entire text up to date. Key reading lists are provided for all topics for those wishing to read about haematology in greater detail. Thanks must also go to the BMJ and in particular Mary Banks, Senior Commissioning Editor, and Sally Carter, Development Editor, who have been key players in the development of the second edition.

I would welcome any comments concerning the book, and perhaps readers may have suggestions for the next edition. I can be contacted at *a.b.provan@qmul.ac.uk*.

1 Iron deficiency anaemia

Drew Provan

Iron deficiency is the commonest cause of anaemia worldwide and is frequently seen in general practice. The anaemia of iron deficiency is caused by defective synthesis of haemoglobin, resulting in red cells that are smaller than normal (microcytic) and contain reduced amounts of haemoglobin (hypochromic).

Iron metabolism

Iron has a pivotal role in many metabolic processes, and the average adult contains 3-5 g of iron, of which two thirds is in the oxygen-carrying molecule haemoglobin.

A normal Western diet provides about 15 mg of iron daily, of which 5-10% is absorbed (~1 mg), principally in the duodenum and upper jejunum, where the acidic conditions help the absorption of iron in the ferrous form. Absorption is helped by the presence of other reducing substances, such as hydrochloric acid and ascorbic acid. The body has the capacity to increase its iron absorption in the face of increased demand—for example, in pregnancy, lactation, growth spurts, and iron deficiency.

Once absorbed from the bowel, iron is transported across the mucosal cell to the blood, where it is carried by the protein transferrin to developing red cells in the bone marrow. Iron stores comprise ferritin, a labile and readily accessible source of iron, and haemosiderin, an insoluble form found predominantly in macrophages.

About 1 mg of iron a day is shed from the body in urine, faeces, sweat, and cells shed from the skin and gastrointestinal tract. Menstrual losses of an additional 20 mg a month and the increased requirements of pregnancy (500-1000 mg) contribute to the higher incidence of iron deficiency in women of reproductive age.

Clinical features of iron deficiency

The symptoms accompanying iron deficiency depend on how rapidly the anaemia develops. In cases of chronic, slow blood loss, the body adapts to the increasing anaemia, and patients can often tolerate extremely low concentrations of haemoglobin—for example, <70 g/l—with remarkably few symptoms. Most patients complain of increasing lethargy and dyspnoea. More unusual symptoms are headaches, tinnitus, and taste disturbance.

On examination, several skin, nail, and other epithelial changes may be seen in chronic iron deficiency. Atrophy of the skin occurs in about a third of patients, and (rarely nowadays) nail changes such as koilonychia (spoon shaped nails) may result in brittle, flattened nails. Patients may also complain of angular stomatitis, in which painful cracks appear at the angle of the mouth, sometimes accompanied by glossitis. Although uncommon, oesophageal and pharyngeal webs can be a feature of iron deficiency anaemia (consider this in middle aged women presenting with dysphagia). These changes are believed to be due to a reduction in the iron-containing enzymes in the epithelium and gastrointestinal tract.

Tachycardia and cardiac failure may occur with severe anaemia irrespective of cause, and in such cases prompt remedial action should be taken.

Table 1.1 Daily dietary iron requirements per 24 hours

Male	1 mg
Adolescence	2-3 mg
Female (reproductive age)	2-3 mg
Pregnancy	3-4 mg
Infancy	1 mg
Maximum bioavailability from normal diet about	4 mg

Box 1.1 Risk factors in development of iron deficiency

- **Age:** infants (especially if history of prematurity); adolescents; postmenopausal women; old age
- **Sex:** increased risk in women
- **Reproduction:** menorrhagia
- **Renal:** haematuria (rarer cause)
- **Gastrointestinal tract:** appetite or weight changes; changes in bowel habit; bleeding from rectum/melaena; gastric or bowel surgery
- **Drug history:** especially aspirin and non-steroidal anti-inflammatories
- **Social history:** diet, especially vegetarians
- **Physiological:** pregnancy; infancy; adolescence; breast feeding; age of weaning

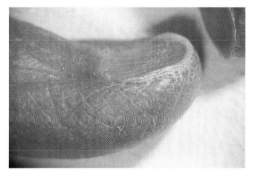

Figure 1.1 Nail changes in iron deficiency anaemia (koilonychia)

Box 1.2 Causes of iron deficiency anaemia

Reproductive system
- Menorrhagia

Gastrointestinal tract
Bleeding
- Oesophagitis
- Oesophageal varices
- Hiatus hernia (ulcerated)
- Peptic ulcer
- Inflammatory bowel disease
- Haemorrhoids (rarely)
- Carcinoma: stomach, colorectal
- Angiodysplasia
- Hereditary haemorrhagic telangiectasia (rare)

Malabsorption
- Coeliac disease
- Atrophic gastritis (also may result *from* iron deficiency)

Physiological
- Growth spurts (especially in premature infants)
- Pregnancy

Dietary
- Vegans
- Elderly

Worldwide commonest cause of iron deficiency is hookworm infection

When iron deficiency is confirmed a full clinical history including leading questions on possible gastrointestinal blood loss or malabsorption (as in, for example, coeliac disease) should be obtained. Menstrual losses should be assessed, and the importance of dietary factors and regular blood donation should not be overlooked.

Diet alone is seldom the sole cause for iron deficiency anaemia in Britain except when it prevents an adequate response to a physiological challenge—as in pregnancy, for example.

Laboratory investigations

A full blood count and film should be taken. These will confirm the anaemia; recognising the indices of iron deficiency is usually straightforward (reduced haemoglobin concentration, reduced mean cell volume, reduced mean cell haemoglobin, reduced mean cell haemoglobin concentration). Some modern analysers will determine the percentage of hypochromic red cells, which may be high before the anaemia develops (it is worth noting that a reduction in haemoglobin concentration is a *late* feature of iron deficiency). The blood film shows microcytic hypochromic red cells. Hypochromic anaemia occurs in other disorders, such as anaemia of chronic disorders and sideroblastic anaemias and in globin synthesis disorders, such as thalassaemia. To help to differentiate the type, further haematinic assays may be necessary. Difficulties in diagnosis arise when more than one type of anaemia is present—for example, iron deficiency and folate deficiency in malabsorption, in a population where thalassaemia is present, or in pregnancy, when the interpretation of red cell indices may be difficult.

Haematinic assays will demonstrate reduced serum ferritin concentration in straightforward iron deficiency. As an acute phase protein, however, the serum ferritin concentration may be normal or even raised in inflammatory or malignant disease.

A prime example of this is found in rheumatoid disease, in which active disease may result in a spuriously raised serum ferritin concentration masking an underlying iron deficiency caused by gastrointestinal bleeding after non-steroidal analgesic treatment. There may also be confusion in liver disease as the liver contains stores of ferritin that are released after hepatocellular damage, leading to raised serum ferritin concentrations. In cases where ferritin estimation is likely to be misleading, the soluble transferrin receptor (sTfR) assay may aid the diagnosis. Transferrin receptors are found on the surface of red cells in greater numbers in iron deficiency; a proportion of receptors are shed into the plasma and can be measured using commercial kits. Unlike the serum ferritin, the sTfR does not rise in inflammatory disorders, and hence can help differentiate between anaemia due to inflammation from iron deficiency.

Diagnostic bone marrow sampling is seldom performed in simple iron deficiency, but if the diagnosis is in doubt a marrow aspirate may be carried out to demonstrate absent bone marrow stores.

When iron deficiency has been diagnosed, the underlying cause should be investigated and treated. Often the history will indicate the likely source of bleeding—for example, menstrual blood loss or gastrointestinal bleeding. If there is no obvious cause, further investigation generally depends on the age and sex of the patient. In male patients and postmenopausal women possible gastrointestinal blood loss is investigated by visualisation of the gastrointestinal tract (endoscopic or barium studies). Faecal occult bloods are of no value in the investigation of iron deficiency.

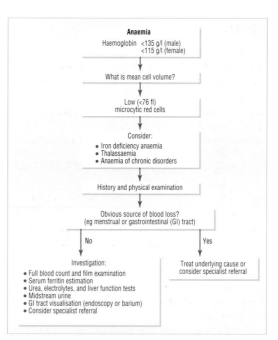

Figure 1.2 Diagnosis and investigation of iron deficiency anaemia

Box 1.3 Investigations in iron deficiency anaemia

- Full clinical history and physical examination
- Full blood count and blood film examination
- Haematinic assays (serum ferritin, vitamin B_{12} folate)
- % hypochromic red cells and soluble transferrin receptor assay (if available)
- Urea and electrolytes, liver function tests
- Fibreoptic and/or barium studies of gastrointestinal tract
- Pelvic ultrasound (females, if indicated)

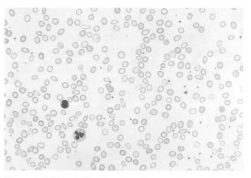

Figure 1.3 Blood film showing changes of iron deficiency anaemia

Table 1.2 Diagnosis of iron deficiency anaemia

Reduced haemoglobin	Men <135 g/l, women <115 g/l
Reduced mean cell volume	<76 fl
Reduced mean cell haemoglobin	29.5 ± 2.5 pg
Reduced mean cell haemoglobin concentration	325 ± 25 g/l
Blood film	Microcytic hypochromic red cells with pencil cells and target cells
Reduced serum ferritin*	Men <10 µg/l, women (postmenopausal) <10 µg/l (premenopausal) <5 µg/l
Elevated % hypochromic red cells (>2%)	
Elevated soluble transferrin receptor level	

*Check with local laboratory for reference ranges

Management

Effective management of iron deficiency relies on (a) the appropriate management of the underlying cause (for example, gastrointestinal or menstrual blood loss) and (b) iron replacement therapy.

Oral iron replacement therapy with gradual replenishment of iron stores and restoration of haemoglobin is the preferred treatment. Oral ferrous salts are the treatment of choice (ferric salts are less well absorbed) and usually take the form of ferrous sulphate 200 mg three times daily (providing 65 mg × 3 = 195 mg elemental iron/day). Alternative preparations include ferrous gluconate and ferrous fumarate. All three compounds, however, are associated with a high incidence of side effects, including nausea, constipation, and diarrhoea. These side effects may be reduced by taking the tablets after meals, but even milder symptoms account for poor compliance with oral iron supplementation. Modified release preparations have been developed to reduce side effects but in practice prove expensive and often release the iron beyond the sites of optimal absorption.

Effective iron replacement therapy should result in a rise in haemoglobin concentration of around 1 g/l per day (about 20 g/l every three weeks), but this varies from patient to patient. Once the haemoglobin concentration is within the normal range, iron replacement should continue for three months to replenish the iron stores.

Failure to respond to oral iron therapy

The main reason for failure to respond to oral iron therapy is poor compliance. However, if the losses (for example, bleeding) exceed the amount of iron absorbed daily, the haemoglobin concentration will not rise as expected; this will also be the case in combined deficiency states.

The presence of underlying inflammation or malignancy may also lead to a poor response to therapy. Finally, an incorrect diagnosis of iron deficiency anaemia should be considered in patients who fail to respond adequately to iron replacement therapy.

Intravenous and intramuscular iron preparations

Parenteral iron may be used when the patient cannot tolerate oral supplements—for example, when patients have severe gastrointestinal side effects or if the losses exceed the daily amount that can be absorbed orally.

Iron sorbitol injection is a complex of iron, sorbitol and citric acid. Treatment consists of a course of deep intramuscular injections. The dosage varies from patient to patient and depends on (a) the initial haemoglobin concentration and (b) body weight. Generally, 10-20 deep intramuscular injections are given over two to three weeks. Apart from being painful, the injections also lead to skin staining at the site of injection and arthralgia, and are best avoided. An intravenous preparation is available (Venofer®) for use in selected cases, and under strict medical supervision, for example, on haematology day unit (risk of anaphylaxis or other reactions).

Alternative treatments

Blood transfusion is not indicated unless the patient has decompensated due to a drop in haemoglobin concentration and needs a more rapid rise in haemoglobin—for example, in cases of worsening angina or severe coexisting pulmonary

Table 1.3 Characteristics of anaemia associated with other disorders

	Iron deficiency	Chronic disorders	Thalassaemia trait (α or β)	Sideroblastic anaemia
Degree of anaemia	Any	Seldom <9.0 g/dl	Mild	Any
MCV	↓	N or ↓	↓ ↓	N or ↓ or ↑
Serum ferritin	↓	N or ↑	N	↑
Soluble transferrin receptor assay	↑	N	↑	N
Marrow iron	Absent	Present	Present	Present

N = norm

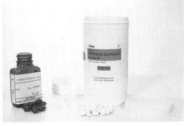

Figure 1.4 Oral iron replacement therapy

Table 1.4 Elemental iron content of various oral iron preparations

Preparation	Amount (mg)	Ferrous iron (mg)
Ferrous fumarate	200	65
Ferrous gluconate	300	35
Ferrous succinate	100	35
Ferrous sulphate	300	60
Ferrous sulphate (dried)	200	65

Box 1.4 Intravenous iron preparations

- Iron dextran no longer available (severe reactions)
- Iron-hydroxide sucrose is currently available in the UK
- Useful in selected cases
- Must be given under close medical supervision and where full resuscitation facilities are available

The rise in haemoglobin concentration is no faster with parenteral iron preparations than with oral iron therapy

disease. In cases of iron deficiency with serious ongoing acute bleeding, blood transfusion may be required.

Prevention

When absorption from the diet is likely to be matched or exceeded by losses, extra sources of iron should be considered—for example, prophylactic iron supplements in pregnancy or after gastrectomy or encouragement of breast feeding or use of formula milk during the first year of life (rather than cows' milk, which is a poor source of iron).

Drs AG Smith and A Amos provided the photographic material and Dr A Odurny provided the radiograph. The source of the detail in the table is the British National Formulary, No 32(Sep), 1995.

Further reading

- Baer AN, Dessypris EN, Krantz SB. The pathogenesis of anemia in rheumatoid arthritis: a clinical and laboratory analysis. *Semin Arthritis Rheum* 1990;19(4):209-23.
- Beguin Y. The soluble transferrin receptor: biological aspects and clinical usefulness as quantitative measure of erythropoiesis. *Haematologica* 1992;77(1):1-10.
- Cook JD, Skikne BS, Baynes RD. Iron deficiency: the global perspective. *Adv Exp Med Biol* 1994;356:219-28.
- DeMaeyer E, Adiels-Tegman M. The prevalence of anaemia in the world. *World Health Stat Q* 1985;38(3):302-16.
- Ferguson BJ, Skikne BS, Simpson KM, Baynes RD, Cook JD. Serum transferrin receptor distinguishes the anemia of chronic disease from iron deficiency anemia. *J Lab Clin Med* 1992;119(4):385-90.
- Finch CA, Huebers HA. Iron metabolism. *Clin Physiol Biochem* 1986;4(1):5-10.
- McIntyre AS, Long RG. Prospective survey of investigations in outpatients referred with iron deficiency anaemia. *Gut* 1993;34(8):1102-7.
- Provan D. Mechanisms and management of iron deficiency anaemia. *Br J Haematol* 1999;105 Suppl 1:19-26.
- Punnonen K, Irjala K, Rajamaki A. Serum transferrin receptor and its ratio to serum ferritin in the diagnosis of iron deficiency. *Blood* 1997;89(3):1052-7.
- Rockey DC, Cello JP. Evaluation of the gastrointestinal tract in patients with iron-deficiency anemia. *N Engl J Med* 1993;329(23):1691-5.
- Windsor CW, Collis JL. Anaemia and hiatus hernia: experience in 450 patients. *Thorax* 1967;22(1):73-8.

2 Macrocytic anaemias

Victor Hoffbrand, Drew Provan

Macrocytosis is a rise in the mean cell volume of the red cells above the normal range (in adults 80-95 fl (femtolitres)). It is detected with a blood count, in which the mean cell volume, as well as other red cell indices, is measured. The mean cell volume is lower in children than in adults, with a normal mean of 70 fl at age 1 year, rising by about 1 fl each year until it reaches adult volumes at puberty.

The causes of macrocytosis fall into two groups: (a) deficiency of vitamin B_{12} (cobalamin) or folate (or rarely abnormalities of their metabolism) in which the bone marrow is megaloblastic, and (b) other causes, in which the bone marrow is usually normoblastic. In this chapter the two groups are considered separately. The reader is then taken through the steps to diagnose the cause of macrocytosis, and subsequently to manage it.

Deficiency of vitamin B_{12} or folate

Vitamin B_{12} deficiency

The body's requirement for vitamin B_{12} is about 1 μg daily. This is amply supplied by a normal Western diet (vitamin B_{12} content 10-30 μg daily) but not by a strict vegan diet, which excludes all animal produce (including milk, eggs, and cheese). Absorption of vitamin B_{12} is through the ileum, facilitated by intrinsic factor, which is secreted by the parietal cells of the stomach. Absorption is limited to 2-3 μg daily.

In Britain, vitamin B_{12} deficiency is usually due to pernicious anaemia, which now accounts for up to 80% of all cases of megaloblastic anaemia. The incidence of the disease is 1;10 000 in northern Europe, and the disease occurs in all races. The underlying mechanism is an autoimmune gastritis that results in achlorhydria and the absence of intrinsic factor. The incidence of pernicious anaemia peaks at age 60; the condition has a female:male incidence of 1.6:1.0 and is more common in those with early greying, blue eyes, and blood group A, and in those with a family history of the disease or of diseases that may be associated with it—for example, vitiligo, myxoedema, Hashimoto's disease, Addison's disease of the adrenal gland, and hypoparathyroidism.

Other causes of vitamin B_{12} deficiency are infrequent in Britain. Veganism is an unusual cause of severe deficiency, as most vegetarians and vegans include some vitamin B_{12} in their diet. Moreover, unlike in pernicious anaemia, the enterohepatic circulation for vitamin B_{12} is intact in vegans, so vitamin B_{12} stores are conserved. Gastric resection and intestinal causes of malabsorption of vitamin B_{12}—for example, ileal resection or the intestinal stagnant loop syndrome—are less common now that abdominal tuberculosis is infrequent and H_2-antagonists have been introduced for treating peptic ulceration, thus reducing the need for gastrectomy.

Folate deficiency

The daily requirement for folate is 100-200 μg, and a normal mixed diet contains about 200-300 μg. Natural folates are largely in the polyglutamate form, and these are absorbed through the upper small intestine after deconjugation and conversion to the monoglutamate 5-methyl tetrahydrofolate.

Body stores are sufficient for only about four months. Folate deficiency may arise because of inadequate dietary

> Megaloblastic bone marrow is exemplified by developing red blood cells that are larger than normal, with nuclei more immature than their cytoplasm. The underlying mechanism is defective DNA synthesis

Box 2.1 Causes of megaloblastic anaemia

Diet
- Vitamin B_{12} deficiency: veganism, poor quality diet
- Folate deficiency: poor quality diet, old age, poverty, synthetic diet without added folic acid, goats' milk

Malabsorption
- Gastric causes of vitamin B_{12} deficiency: pernicious anaemia, congenital intrinsic factor deficiency or abnormality gastrectomy
- Intestinal causes of vitamin B_{12} deficiency: stagnant loop, congenital selective malabsorption, ileal resection, Crohn's disease
- Intestinal causes of folate deficiency: gluten-induced enteropathy, tropical sprue, jejunal resection

Increased cell turnover
- Folate deficiency: pregnancy, prematurity, chronic haemolytic anaemia (such as sickle cell anaemia), extensive inflammatory and malignant diseases

Renal loss
- Folate deficiency: congestive cardiac failure, dialysis

Drugs
- Folate deficiency: anticonvulsants, sulphasalazine

Defects of vitamin B_{12} metabolism—eg transcobalamin II deficiency, nitrous oxide anaesthesia—or of folate metabolism (such as methotrexate treatment), or rare inherited defects of DNA synthesis may all cause megaloblastic anaemia

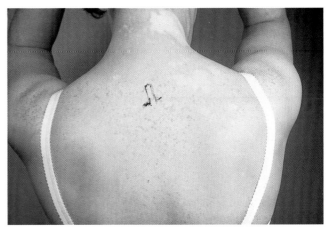

Figure 2.1 Patient with vitiligo on neck and back

intake, malabsorption (especially gluten-induced enteropathy), or excessive use as proliferating cells degrade folate. Deficiency in pregnancy may be due partly to inadequate diet, partly to transfer of folate to the fetus, and partly to increased folate degradation.

Consequences of vitamin B₁₂ or folate deficiencies

Megaloblastic anaemia—Clinical features include pallor and jaundice. The onset is gradual, and a severely anaemic patient may present in congestive heart failure or only when an infection supervenes. The blood film shows oval macrocytes and hypersegmented neutrophil nuclei (with six or more lobes). In severe cases, the white cell count and platelet count also fall (pancytopenia). The bone marrow shows characteristic megaloblastic erythroblasts and giant metamyelocytes (granulocyte precursors). Biochemically, there is an increase in plasma of unconjugated bilirubin and serum lactic dehydrogenase, with, in severe cases, an absence of haptoglobins and presence in urine of haemosiderin. These changes, including jaundice, are due to increased destruction of red cell precursors in the marrow (ineffective erythropoiesis).

Vitamin B₁₂ neuropathy—A minority of patients with vitamin B₁₂ deficiency develop a neuropathy due to symmetrical damage to the peripheral nerves and posterior and lateral columns of the spinal cord, the legs being more affected than the arms. Psychiatric abnormalities and visual disturbance may also occur. Men are more commonly affected than women. The neuropathy may occur in the absence of anaemia. Psychiatric changes and at most a mild peripheral neuropathy may be ascribed to folate deficiency.

Neural tube defects—Folic acid supplements in pregnancy have been shown to reduce the incidence of neural tube defects (spina bifida, encephalocoele, and anencephaly) in the fetus and may also reduce the incidence of cleft palate and hare lip. No clear relation exists between the incidence of these defects and folate deficiency in the mother, although the lower the maternal red cell folate (and serum vitamin B₁₂) concentrations even within the normal range, the more likely neural tube defects are to occur in the fetus. An underlying mechanism in a minority of cases is a genetic defect in folate metabolism, a mutation in the enzyme 5, 10 methylenetetra hydrofolate reductase.

Gonadal dysfunction—Deficiency of either vitamin B₁₂ or folate may cause sterility, which is reversible with appropriate vitamin supplementation.

Epithelial cell changes—Glossitis and other epithelial surfaces may show cytological abnormalities.

Cardiovascular disease—Raised serum homocysteine concentrations have been associated with arterial obstruction (myocardial infarct, peripheral vascular disease or stroke) and venous thrombosis. Trials are under way to determine whether folic acid supplementation reduces the incidence of these vascular diseases.

Other causes of macrocytosis

The most common cause of macrocytosis in Britain is alcohol. Fairly small quantities of alcohol—for example, two gin and tonics or half a bottle of wine a day—especially in women, may cause a rise of mean cell volume to >100 fl, typically without anaemia or any detectable change in liver function.

The mechanism for the rise in mean cell volume is uncertain. In liver disease the volume may rise due to excessive lipid deposition on red cell membranes, and the rise is particularly pronounced in liver disease caused by alcohol.

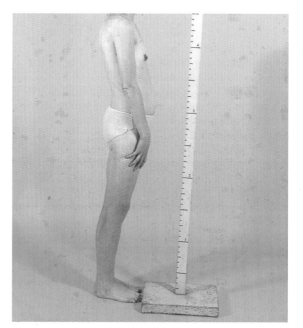

Figure 2.2 Patient with celiac disease: underweight and low stature

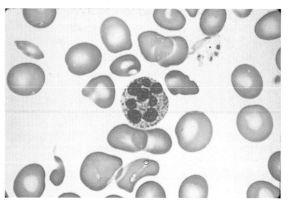

Figure 2.3 Blood film in vitamin B₁₂ deficiency showing macrocytic red cells and a hypersegmented neutrophil

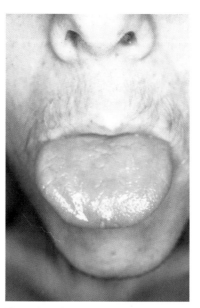

Figure 2.4 Glossitis due to vitamin B₁₂ deficiency

A modest rise in mean cell volume is found in severe thyroid deficiency.

In other causes of macrocytosis, other haematological abnormalities are usually present—in myelodysplasia (a frequent cause of macrocytosis in elderly people) there are usually quantitative or qualitative changes in the white cells and platelets in the blood. In aplastic anaemia, pancytopenia is present; pure red cell aplasia may also cause macrocytosis. Changes in plasma proteins—presence of a paraprotein (as in myeloma)—may cause a rise in mean cell volume without macrocytes being present in the blood film. Physiological causes of macrocytosis are pregnancy and the neonatal period. Drugs that affect DNA synthesis—for example, hydroxyurea and azathioprine—can cause macrocytosis with or without megaloblastic changes. Finally, a rare, benign familial type of macrocytosis has been described.

Diagnosis

Biochemical assays
The most widely used screening tests for the deficiencies are the serum vitamin B_{12} and folate assays. A low serum concentration implies deficiency, but a subnormal serum concentration may occur in the absence of pronounced body deficiency—for example, in pregnancy (vitamin B_{12}) and with recent poor dietary intake (folate).

Red cell folate can also be used to screen for folate deficiency; a low concentration usually implies appreciable depletion of body folate, but the concentration also falls in severe vitamin B_{12} deficiency, so it is more difficult to interpret the significance of a low red cell than serum folate concentration in patients with megaloblastic anaemia. Moreover, if the patient has received a recent blood transfusion the red cell folate concentration will partly reflect the folate concentration of the transfused red cells.

Specialist investigations
Assays of serum homocysteine (raised in vitamin B_{12} or folate deficiency) or methylmalonic acid (raised in vitamin B_{12} deficiency) are used in some specialised laboratories. Serum homocysteine levels are also raised in renal failure, with certain drugs, e.g. corticosteroids, and increase with age and smoking.

Autoantibodies
For patients with vitamin B_{12} or folate deficiency it is important to establish the underlying cause. In pernicious anaemia, intrinsic factor antibodies are present in plasma in 50% of patients and in parietal cell antibodies in 90%. Antigliadin, anti-endomysial and antireticulin antibodies are usually positive in gluten-induced enteropathy.

Other investigations
A bone marrow examination is usually performed to confirm megaloblastic anaemia. It is also required for the diagnosis of myelodysplasia, aplastic anaemia, myeloma, or other marrow disorders associated with macrocytosis.

Radioactive vitamin B_{12} absorption studies—for example, Schilling test—show impaired absorption of the vitamin in pernicious anaemia; this can be corrected by giving intrinsic factor. In patients with an intestinal lesion, however, absorption of vitamin B_{12} cannot be corrected with intrinsic factor. Human intrinsic factor is no longer licensed for this test because of concern about transmission of prion disease.

Endoscopy should be performed to confirm atrophic gastritis and exclude gastric carcinoma or gastric polyps, which

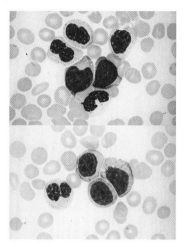

> **Box 2.2 Other causes of macrocytosis***
> - Alcohol
> - Liver disease
> - Hypothyroidism
> - Reticulocytosis
> - Aplastic anaemia
> - Red cell aplasia
> - Myelodysplasia
> - Cytotoxic drugs
> - Paraproteinaemia (such as myeloma)
> - Pregnancy
> - Neonatal period
>
> *These are usually associated with a normoblastic marrow

Figure 2.5 Bone marrow aspirate in myelodysplasia showing characteristic dysplastic neutrophils with bilobed nuclei

> **Box 2.3 Investigations that may be needed in patients with macrocytosis**
> - Serum vitamin B_{12} assay
> - Serum and red cell folate assays
> - Liver and thyroid function
> - Reticulocyte count
> - Serum protein electrophoresis
> - For vitamin B_{12} deficiency: serum parietal cell and intrinsic factor antibodies, radioactive vitamin B_{12} absorption with and without intrinsic factor (Schilling test), possibly serum gastrin concentration
> - For folate deficiency: antigliadin, anti-endomysial and antireticulin antibodies
> - Consider bone marrow examination for megaloblastic changes suggestive of vitamin B_{12} or folate deficiency, or alternative diagnoses—eg myelodysplasia, aplastic anaemia, myeloma
> - Endoscopy—gastric biopsy (vitamin B_{12} deficiency); duodenal biopsy (folate deficiency)
> - Serum antigliadin and anti-endomysial antibodies

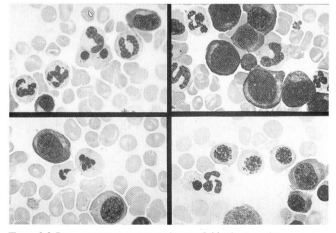

Figure 2.6 Bone marrow appearances in megaloblastic anaemia: developing red cells are larger than normal, with nuclei that are immature relative to their cytoplasm (nuclear:cytoplasmic asynchrony)

are two to three times more common in patients with pernicious anaemia than in age and sex matched controls.

If folate deficiency is diagnosed, it is important to assess dietary folate intake and to exclude gluten induced enteropathy by tests for serum antigliadin and anti-endomysial antibodies, endoscopy and duodenal biopsy. The deficiency is common in patients with diseases of increased cell turnover who also have a poor diet.

Treatment

Vitamin B_{12} deficiency is treated initially by giving the patient six injections of hydroxo-cobalamin 1 mg at intervals of about three to four days, followed by four such injections a year for life. For patients undergoing total gastrectomy or ileal resection it is sensible to start the maintenance injections from the time of operation. For vegans, less frequent injections—for example, one or two a year—may be sufficient, and the patient should be advised to eat foods to which vitamin B_{12} has been added, such as certain fortified breads or other foods.

Folate deficiency is treated with folic acid, usually 5 mg daily orally for four months, which is continued only if the underlying cause cannot be corrected. As prophylaxis against folate deficiency in patients with a severe haemolytic anaemia— such as sickle cell anaemia—5 mg folic acid once weekly is probably sufficient. Vitamin B_{12} deficiency must be excluded in all patients starting folic acid treatment at these doses as such treatment may correct the anaemia in vitamin B_{12} deficiency but allow neurological disease to develop.

Further reading

- Carmel R. Current concepts in cobalamin deficiency. *Annu Rev Med* 2000;51:357-75.
- Clarke R, Smith AD, Jobst KA, Refsum H, Sutton L, Ueland PM. Folate, vitamin B_{12}, and serum total homocysteine levels in confirmed Alzheimer disease. *Arch Neurol* 1998;55(11):1449-55.
- Haynes WG. Homocysteine and atherosclerosis: potential mechanisms and clinical implications. *Proc R Coll Phys Edinb* 2000;30:114-22.
- Jacques PF, Selhub J, Bostom AG, Wilson PW, Rosenberg IH. The effect of folic acid fortification on plasma folate and total homocysteine concentrations. *N Engl J Med* 1999;340(19):1449-54.
- Lindenbaum J, Allen RH. Clinical spectrum and diagnosis of folate deficiency. In: Bailey LB. Folate in health and disease. New York: Marcel Dekker 1995;pp43-73.
- Mills JL. Fortification of foods with folic acid—how much is enough? *N Engl J Med* 2000;342(19):1442-5.
- Perry DJ. Hyperhomocysteinaemia. *Baillieres Best Pract Res Clin Haematol* 1999;12(3):451-77.
- Wickramasinghe SN. Morphology, biology and biochemistry of cobalamin- and folate-deficient bone marrow cells. *Baillieres Clin Haematol* 1995;8(3):441-59.

Table 2.1 Results of absorption tests of radioactive vitamin B_{12}

	Dose of vitamin B_{12} given alone	Dose of vitamin B_{12} given with intrinsic factor[†]
Vegan	Normal	Normal
Pernicious anaemia or gastrectomy	Low	Normal
Ileal resection	Low	Low
Intestinal blind-loop syndrome	Low[*]	Low[*]

[*]Corrected by antibodies.
[†]Human intrinsic factor no longer licensed for this test because of concern about prion transmission

Box 2.4 Preventing folate deficiency in pregnancy

- As prophylaxis against folate deficiency in pregnancy, daily doses of folic acid 400 µg are usual
- Larger doses are not recommended as they could mask megaloblastic anaemia due to vitamin B_{12} deficiency and thus allow B_{12} neuropathy to develop
- As neural tube defects occur by the 28th day of pregnancy, it is advisable for a woman's daily folate intake to be increased by 400 µg/day at the time of conception
- The US Food and Drugs Administration announced in 1996 that specified grain products (including most enriched breads, flours, cornmeal, rice, noodles, and macaroni) will be required to be fortified with folic acid to levels ranging from 0.43 mg to 1.5 mg per pound (453 g) of product. Fortification of flour with folic acid is currently under discussion in the UK
- For mothers who have already had an infant with a neural tube defect, larger doses of folic acid—eg 5 mg daily—are recommended before and during subsequent pregnancy

The illustration of the bone marrow (Figure 2.6) is reproduced with permission from *Clinical haematology* (AV Hoffbrand, J Pettit), 3rd ed, St Louis: CV Mosby, 2000.

3   The hereditary anaemias

David J Weatherall

Hereditary anaemias include disorders of the structure or synthesis of haemoglobin; deficiencies of enzymes that provide the red cell with energy or protect it from chemical damage; and abnormalities of the proteins of the red cell's membrane. Inherited diseases of haemoglobin—haemoglobinopathies—are by far the most important.

The structure of human haemoglobin (Hb) changes during development. By the 12th week embryonic haemoglobin is replaced by fetal haemoglobin (Hb F), which is slowly replaced after birth by the adult haemoglobins, Hb A and Hb A_2. Each type of haemoglobin consists of two different pairs of peptide chains; Hb A has the structure $\alpha_2\beta_2$ (namely, two α chains plus two β chains), Hb A_2 has the structure of $\alpha_2\delta_2$, and Hb F, $\alpha_2\gamma_2$.

The haemoglobinopathies consist of structural haemoglobin variants (the most important of which are the sickling disorders) and thalassaemias (hereditary defects of the synthesis of either the α or β globin chains).

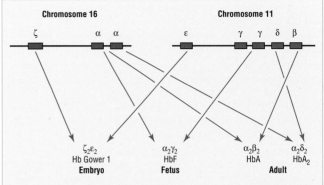

Figure 3.1 Simplified representation of the genetic control of human haemoglobin. Because α chains are shared by both fetal and adult Hb, mutations of the α globin genes affect Hb production in both fetal and adult life; diseases that are due to defective β globin production are only manifest after birth when Hb A replace Hb F

The sickling disorders

Classification and inheritance

The common sickling disorders consist of the homozygous state for the sickle cell gene—that is, sickle cell anaemia (Hb SS)—and the compound heterozygous state for the sickle cell gene and that for either Hb C (another β chain variant) or β thalassaemia (termed Hb SC disease or sickle cell β thalassaemia). The sickle cell mutation results in a single amino acid substitution in the β globin chain; heterozygotes have one normal (β^A) and one affected β chain (β^S) gene and produce about 60% Hb A and 40% Hb S; homozygotes produce mainly Hb S with small amounts of Hb F. Compound heterozygotes for Hb S and Hb C produce almost equal amounts of each variant, whereas those who inherit the sickle cell gene from one parent and β thalassaemia from the other make predominantly sickle haemoglobin.

Pathophysiology

The amino acid substitution in the β globin chain causes red cell sickling during deoxygenation, leading to increased rigidity and aggregation in the microcirculation. These changes are reflected by a haemolytic anaemia and episodes of tissue infarction.

Geographical distribution

The sickle cell gene is spread widely throughout Africa and in countries with African immigrant populations; some Mediterranean countries; the Middle East; and parts of India. Screening should not be restricted to people of African origin.

Clinical features

Sickle cell carriers are not anaemic and have no clinical abnormalities. Patients with sickle cell anaemia have a haemolytic anaemia, with haemoglobin concentration 60-100 g/l and a high reticulocyte count; the blood film shows polychromasia and sickled erythrocytes.

Patients adapt well to their anaemia, and it is the vascular occlusive or sequestration episodes ("crises") that pose the main threat. Crises take several forms. The commonest, called the painful crisis, is associated with widespread bone pain and is usually self-limiting. More serious and life threatening crises

---

Box 3.1 Sickling syndromes

- Hb SS (sickle cell anaemia)
- Hb SC disease
- Hb S/β^+ thalassaemia
- Hb S/β^0 thalassaemia
- Hb SD disease

Box 3.2 Sickle cell trait (Hb A and Hb S)

- Less than half the Hb in each red cell is Hb S
- Occasional renal papillary necrosis
- Inability to concentrate the urine (older individuals)
- Red cells do not sickle unless oxygen saturations <40% (rarely reached in venous blood)
- Painful crises and splenic infarction have been reported in severe hypoxia—such as unpressurised aircraft, anaesthesia

Sickling is more severe where Hb S is present with another β globin chain abnormality—such as Hb S and Hb C (Hb SC) or Hb S and Hb D (Hb SD)

Box 3.3 Sickle cell anaemia (homozygous Hb S)

- Anaemia (Hb 60-100 g/l): symptoms milder than expected as Hb S has reduced oxygen affinity (that is, gives up oxygen to tissues more easily)
- Sickled cells may be present in blood film: sickling occurs at oxygen tensions found in venous blood; cyclical sickling episodes
- Reticulocytes: raised to 10-20%
- Red cells contain ≥80% Hb S (rest is maily fetal Hb)
- Variable haemolysis
- Hand and foot syndrome (dactylitis)
- Intermittent episodes, or crises, characterised by bone pain, worsening anaemia, or pulmonary or neurological disease
- Chronic leg ulcers
- Gall stones

include the sequestration of red cells into the lung or spleen, strokes, or red cell aplasia associated with parvovirus infections.

Diagnosis
Sickle cell anaemia should be suspected in any patient of an appropriate racial group with a haemolytic anaemia. It can be confirmed by a sickle cell test, although this does not distinguish between heterozygotes and homozygotes. A definitive diagnosis requires haemoglobin electrophoresis and the demonstration of the sickle cell trait in both parents.

Prevention and treatment
Pregnant women in at-risk racial groups should be screened in early pregnancy and, if the woman and her partner are carriers, should be offered either prenatal or neonatal diagnosis. As soon as the diagnosis is established babies should receive penicillin daily and be immunised against *Streptococcus pneumoniae*, *Haemophilus influenzae* type b, and *Neisseria meningitidis*. Parents should be warned to seek medical advice on any suspicion of infection. Painful crises should be managed with adequate analgesics, hydration, and oxygen. The patient should be observed carefully for a source of infection and a drop in haemoglobin concentration. Pulmonary sequestration crises require urgent exchange transfusion together with oxygen therapy. Strokes should be treated with a transfusion; there is good evidence now that they can be prevented by regular surveillance of cerebral blood flow by Doppler examination and prophylactic transfusion. There is also good evidence that the frequency of painful crises can be reduced by maintaining patients on hydroxyurea, although because of the uncertainty about the long term effects of this form of therapy, it should be restricted to adults or, if it is used in children, this should be only for a short period. Aplastic crises require urgent blood transfusion. Splenic sequestration crises require transfusion and, because they may recur, splenectomy is advised.

Sickling variants
Hb SC disease is characterised by a mild anaemia and fewer crises. Important microvascular complications, however, include retinal damage and blindness, aseptic necrosis of the femoral heads, and recurrent haematuria. The disease is occasionally complicated by pulmonary embolic disease, particularly during and after pregnancy; these episodes should be treated by immediate exchange transfusion. Patients with Hb SC should have annual ophthalmological surveillance; the retinal vessel proliferation can be controlled with laser treatment.

> **Box 3.4 Complications of sickle cell disease**
> - Hand and foot syndrome: seen in infancy; painful swelling of digits
> - Painful crises: later in life; generalised bone pain; precipitated by cold, dehydration but often no cause found; self limiting over a few days
> - Aplastic crisis: marrow temporarily hypoplastic; may follow parvovirus infection; profound anaemia; reduced reticulocyte count
> - Splenic sequestration crisis: common in infancy; progressive anaemia; enlargement of spleen
> - Hepatic sequestration crisis: similar to splenic crisis but with sequestration of red cells in liver
> - Lung or brain syndromes: sickling of red cells in pulmonary or cerebral circulation and endothelial damage to cerebral vessels in cerebral circulation
> - Infections: particularly *Streptococcus pneumoniae* and *Haemophilus influenzae*
> - Gall stones
> - Progressive renal failure
> - Chronic leg ulcers
> - Recurrent priapism
> - Aseptic necrosis of humoral/femoral head
> - Chronic osteomyelitis: sometimes due to *Salmonella typhi*

> **Box 3.5 Treatment of major complications of sickle cell disease**
> - Hand and foot syndrome: hydration; paracetamol
> - Painful crises: hydration; analgesia (including graded intravenous analgesics); oxygen (check arterial blood gases); blood cultures; antibiotics
> - Pulmonary infiltrates: especially with deterioration in arterial gases, falling platelet count and/or haemoglobin concentration suggesting lung syndrome requires urgent exchange blood transfusion to reduce Hb S level together with oxygenation
> - Splenic sequestration crisis: transfusion; splenectomy to prevent recurrence
> - Neurological symptoms: immediate exchange transfusion followed by long term transfusion
> - Prevention of crises: ongoing trials of cytotoxic agent hydroxyurea show that it raises Hb F level and ameliorates frequency and severity of crises; long term effects unknown

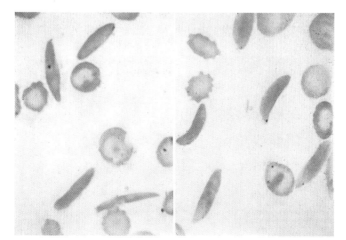

Figure 3.2 Peripheral blood film from patient with sickle cell anaemia showing sickled erythrocytes

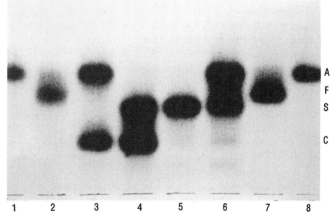

Figure 3.3 Haemoglobin electrophoresis showing (1) normal, (2) newborn, (3) Hb C trait (A-C), (4) Hb SC disease (SC), (5) sickle cell disease (SS), (6) sickle cell trait (A-S), (7) newborn, (8) normal

The management of the symptomatic forms of sickle cell β thalassaemia is similar to that of sickle cell anaemia.

The thalassaemias

Classification

The thalassaemias are classified as α or β thalassaemias, depending on which pair of globin chains is synthesised inefficiently. Rarer forms affect both β and δ chain production—δβ thalassaemias.

Distribution

The disease is broadly distributed throughout parts of Africa, the Mediterranean region, the Middle East, the Indian subcontinent, and South East Asia, and it occurs sporadically in all racial groups. Like sickle cell anaemia, it is thought to be common because carriers have been protected against malaria.

Inheritance

The β thalassaemias result from over 150 different mutations of the β globin genes, which reduce the output of β globin chains, either completely (β° thalassaemia) or partially (β⁺ thalassaemia). They are inherited like sickle cell anaemia; carrier parents have a one in four chance of having a homozygous child. The genetics of the α thalassaemias is more complicated because normal people have two α globin genes on each of their chromosomes 16. If both are lost (α° thalassaemia) no α globin chains are made, whereas if only one of the pair is lost (α⁺ thalassaemia) the output of α globin chains is reduced. Impaired α globin production leads to excess γ or β chains that form unstable and physiologically useless tetramers, γ₄ (Hb Bart's) and β₄ (Hb H). The homozygous state for α° thalassaemia results in the Hb Bart's hydrops syndrome, whereas the inheritance of α° and α⁺ thalassaemia produces Hb H disease.

The β thalassaemias

Heterozygotes for β thalassaemia are asymptomatic, have hypochromic microcytic red cells with a low mean cell haemoglobin and mean cell volume, and have a mean Hb A₂ level of about twice normal. Homozygotes, or those who have inherited a different β thalassaemia gene from both parents, usually develop severe anaemia in the first year of life. This results from a deficiency of β globin chains; excess α chains precipitate in the red cell precursors leading to their damage, either in the bone marrow or the peripheral blood. Hypertrophy of the ineffective bone marrow leads to skeletal changes, and there is variable hepatosplenomegaly. The Hb F level is always raised. If these children are transfused, the marrow is "switched off", and growth and development may be normal. However, they accumulate iron and may die later from damage to the myocardium, pancreas, or liver. They are also prone to infection and folic acid deficiency. Milder forms of β thalassaemia (thalassaemia intermedia), although not transfusion dependent, are sometimes associated with similar bone changes, anaemia, leg ulcers, and delayed development.

The α thalassaemias

The Hb Bart's hydrops fetalis syndrome is characterised by the stillbirth of a severely oedematous (hydropic) fetus in the second half of pregnancy. Hb H disease is associated with a moderately severe haemolytic anaemia. The carrier states for α° thalassaemia or the homozygous state for α⁺ thalassaemia result in a mild hypochromic anaemia with normal Hb A₂ levels. They can only be distinguished with certainty by DNA analysis in a

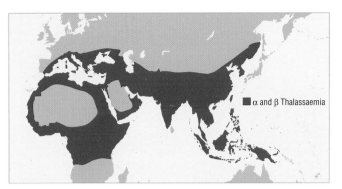

Figure 3.4 Distribution of the thalassaemias (red area)

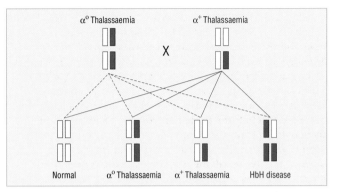

Figure 3.5 Inheritance of Hb disease (open boxes represent normal α globin genes and red boxes, deleted α globin genes)

Box 3.6 β Thalassaemia trait (heterozygous carrier)

- Mild hypochromic microcytic anaemia
    Haemoglobin 90-110 g/l
    Mean cell volume 50-70 fl
    Mean corpuscular haemoglobin 20-22 pg
- No clinical features, patients asymptomatic
- Often diagnosed on routine blood count
- Raised Hb A₂ level

Box 3.7 β Thalassaemia major (homozygous β thalassaemia)

- Severe anaemia
- Blood film
    Pronounced variation in red cell size and shape
    Pale (hypochromic) red cells
    Target cells
    Basophilic stippling
    Nucleated red cells
    Moderately raised reticulocyte count
- Infants are well at birth but develop anaemia in first few months of life when switch occurs from γ to β globin chains
- Progressive splenomegaly; iron loading; proneness to infection

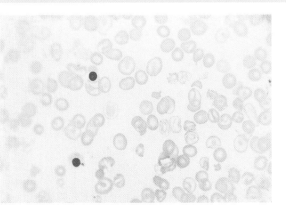

Figure 3.6 Peripheral blood film in homozygous β thalassaemia showing pronounced hypochromia and anisocytosis with nucleated red blood cells

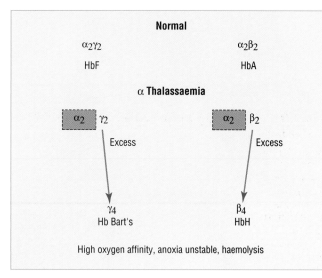

Figure 3.7 Pathophysiology of α thalassaemia

specialised laboratory. In addition to the distribution mentioned above, α thalassaemia is also seen in European populations in association with mental retardation; the molecular pathology is quite different to the common inherited forms of the condition. There are two major forms of α thalassaemia associated with mental retardation (ATR); one is encoded on chromosome 16 (ATR-16) and the other on the X chromosome (ATRX). ATR-16 is usually associated with mild mental retardation and is due to loss of the α globin genes together with other genetic material from the end of the short arm of chromosome 16. ATRX is associated with more severe mental retardation and a variety of skeletal deformities and is encoded by a gene on the X chromosome which is expressed widely in different tissues during different stages of development. These conditions should be suspected in any infant or child with retarded development who has the haematological picture of a mild α thalassaemia trait.

Prevention and treatment
As β thalassaemia is easily identified in heterozygotes, pregnant women of appropriate racial groups should be screened; if a woman is found to be a carrier, her partner should be tested and the couple counselled. Prenatal diagnosis by chorionic villus sampling can be carried out between the 9th and 13th weeks of pregnancy. If diagnosis is established, the patients should be treated by regular blood transfusion with surveillance for hepatitis C and related infections.

To prevent iron overload, overnight infusions of desferrioxamine together with vitamin C should be started, and the patient's serum ferritin, or better, hepatic iron concentrations, should be monitored; complications of desferrioxamine include infections with *Yersinia* spp, retinal and acoustic nerve damage, and reduction in growth associated with calcification of the vertebral discs. The place of the oral chelating agent deferiprone is still under evaluation. It is now clear that it does not maintain iron balance in approximately 50% of patients and its long term toxicity remains to be evaluated by adequate controlled trials. It is known to cause neutropenia and transient arthritis. Current studies are directed at assessing its value in combination with desferrioxamine. Bone marrow transplantation—if appropriate HLA-DR matched siblings are available—may carry a good prognosis if carried out early in life. Treatment with agents designed to raise the production of Hb F is still at the experimental stage.

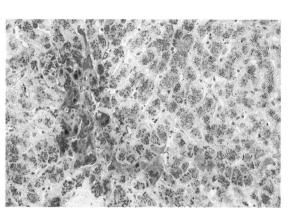

Figure 3.8 Liver biopsy from patient with β thalassaemia showing pronounced iron accumulation

In β thalassaemia and Hb H disease progressive splenomegaly or increasing blood requirements, or both, indicate that splenectomy may be beneficial. Patients who undergo splenectomy should be vaccinated against *S pneumoniae*, *H influenzae*, and *N meningitidis* preoperatively and should receive a maintenance dose of oral penicillin indefinitely.

Red cell enzyme defects

Red cells have two main metabolic pathways, one burning glucose anaerobically to produce energy, the other generating reduced glutathione to protect against injurious oxidants. Many inherited enzyme defects have been described. Some of those of the energy pathway—for example, pyruvate kinase deficiency—cause haemolytic anaemia; any child with this kind of anaemia from birth should be referred to a centre capable of analysing the major red cell enzymes.

Glucose-6-phosphate dehydrogenase deficiency (G6PD) involves the protective pathway. It affects millions of people worldwide, mainly the same racial groups as are affected by the thalassaemias. Glucose-6-phosphate dehydrogenase deficiency is sex linked and affects males predominantly. It causes neonatal jaundice, sensitivity to fava beans (broad beans), and haemolytic responses to oxidant drugs.

Red cell membrane defects

The red cell membrane is a complex sandwich of proteins that are required to maintain the integrity of the cell. There are many inherited defects of the membrane proteins, some of which cause haemolytic anaemia. Hereditary spherocytosis is due to a structural change that makes the cells more leaky. It is particularly important to identify this disease because it can be "cured" by splenectomy. There are many rare inherited varieties of elliptical or oval red cells, some associated with chronic haemolysis and response to splenectomy. A child with a chronic haemolytic anaemia with abnormally shaped red cells should always be referred for expert advice.

Other hereditary anaemias

Other anaemias with an important inherited component include Fanconi's anaemia (hypoplastic anaemia with skeletal deformities), Blackfan-Diamond anaemia (red cell aplasia), and several forms of congenital dyserythropoietic anaemia.

Box 3.10 Drugs causing haemolysis in patients with G6PD deficiency

Antimalarials
Primiquine
Pamaquine

Analgesics*
Phenacetin
Acetyl salicylic acid

Others
Sulphonamides
Nalidixic acid
Dapsone

*Probably only at high doses

Further reading
- Ballas SK. Sickle cell disease: clinical management. *Clin Haematol* 1998;11:185-214.
- Luzzatto L, Gordon-Smith EC. Hereditary haemolytic anaemia. In: Hoffbrand AV, Lewis SM, Tuddenham GD, eds. *Postgraduate haematology*. Oxford: Butterworth-Heinemann, 1999, pp144-163.
- Steinberg MH. Pathophysiology of sickle cell disease. *Clin Haematol* 1998;11:163-84.
- Steinberg MH, Forget BG, Higgs DR, Nagel RL. *Disorders of haemoglobin*. Cambridge: Cambridge University Press, 2001.
- Weatherall DJ. The thalassemias. In: Stamatayonnopoulos G, Perlmutter RM, Marjerus PW, Varmus H, eds. *Molecular basis of blood diseases*, 3rd edn. Philadelphia: WB Saunders, 2001, pp186-226.
- Weatherall DJ, Clegg JB. *The thalassemia syndromes*, 4th edn. Oxford: Blackwell Science, 2001.
- Weatherall DJ, Clegg JB, Higgs DR, Wood WG. The hemoglobinopathies. In: Scriver CR, Beaudet AL, Sly WS, Valle D, Childs B, Vogelstein B, eds. *The metabolic and molecular bases of inherited disease*, 8th edn. New York: McGraw-Hill, 2001, pp4571-636.

4 Polycythaemia, essential thrombocythaemia, and myelofibrosis

George S Vassiliou, Anthony R Green

Polycythaemia vera, essential thrombocythaemia and idiopathic myelofibrosis are all clonal disorders originating from a single aberrant neoplastic stem cell in the bone marrow. They are generally diseases of middle or older age and have features in common, including a potential for transforming to acute leukaemia. Myelofibrosis may arise de novo or result from progression of polycythaemia vera or essential thrombocythaemia. Treatment of polycythaemia vera and essential thrombocythaemia can greatly influence prognosis, hence the importance of diagnosing these rare disorders early. They need to be distinguished from other types of polycythaemia (secondary polycythaemia, apparent polycythaemia) and other causes of a raised platelet count (secondary or reactive thrombocytosis), whose prognosis and treatment are different.

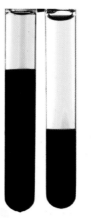

Figure 4.1 Raised PCV in a patient with true polycythaemia secondary to congenital cyanotic heart disease (left) compared to a blood sample from a person with a normal PCV (right)

Polycythaemia

An elevation in packed cell volume (PCV), rather than a raised haemoglobin concentration, defines polycythaemia. A raised packed cell volume (>0.51 in males, >0.48 in females) needs to be confirmed on a specimen taken without prolonged venous stasis (tourniquet). Patients with a persistently raised packed cell volume should be referred to a haematologist for measurement of red cell mass by radionuclide labelling of the red cells. Red cell mass is best expressed as the percentage difference between the measured value and that predicted from the patient's height and weight (derived from tables).

Red cell mass measurements more than 25% above the predicted value constitute *true or absolute polycythaemia*, which can be classified into aetiological categories. When the packed cell volume is raised but the red cell mass is not, the condition is known as *apparent or relative polycythaemia* and is secondary to a reduction in plasma volume.

Polycythaemia vera

Presentation can be incidental but is classically associated with a history of occlusive vascular lesions (stroke, transient ischaemic attack, ischaemic digits), headache, mental clouding, facial redness, itching, abnormal bleeding, or gout.

Initial laboratory investigations—A raised white cell count ($>10 \times 10^9/1$ neutrophils) or a raised platelet count ($>400 \times 10^9/1$) suggest primary polycythaemia, especially if both are raised in the absence of an obvious cause, such as infection or carcinoma. Serum ferritin concentration should be determined as iron deficiency may mask a raised packed cell volume, resulting in a missed diagnosis.

Specialist investigations—Red cell mass should be determined to confirm absolute polycythaemia, and secondary polycythaemia should be excluded. Most patients with primary polycythaemia have a low serum erythropoietin concentration. If the spleen is not palpable then splenic sizing (ultrasonography) should be performed to look for enlargement. Bone marrow cytogenetic analysis may reveal an acquired chromosomal abnormality which would favour a primary marrow disorder such as polycythaemia vera. Erythroid

> **Box 4.1 Classification of true polycythaemias**
> **Familial/inherited**
> * Mutant erythropoietin receptor
> * High oxygen affinity haemoglobin
>
> **Acquired**
> *Primary*
> * Polycythaemia vera
>
> *Secondary*
> * Hypoxia
>   cardiac
>   pulmonary
>   central
> * Ectopic erythropoietin
>   renal disease
>   neoplasms

> **Palpable splenomegaly is present in less than half the patients with polycythaemia vera, but when present it strongly favours this diagnosis over other polycythaemias**

> **Box 4.2 Investigations of a raised packed cell volume**
> * Red cell mass estimation
>
> *If red cell mass is elevated or equivocal then proceed with:*
> * Arterial blood oxygen saturation
> * Abdominal ultrasound
> * Bone marrow aspirate, trephine and cytogenetic examination
> * Serum erythropoietin level
> * Culture blood for spontaneous erythroid colonies

colony growth from blood or bone marrow in the absence of added erythropoietin culture from peripheral blood would support the diagnosis. No single pathognomonic test exists and the diagnosis is best made using a diagnostic algorithm (opposite).

Treatment—Traditional treatment using the marrow suppressant effect of radioactive phosphorus (^{32}P) has been superseded because of the additional risk of inducing malignancies such as acute leukaemia in later life. Repeated venesection to maintain the packed cell volume at <0.45 has become the mainstay of treatment. At this volume the risk of thrombotic episodes is much reduced. Venesection has to be frequent at first but is eventually needed only every 6-10 weeks in most patients. If thrombocytosis is present, concurrent therapy to maintain the platelet count to $<400 \times 10^9/l$ is necessary. Hydroxyurea (0.5-1.5 g daily) is recommended for this purpose and is not thought to have a pronounced leukaemogenic potential. Some use interferon α in preference to hydroxyurea in younger patients, as this drug is not thought to increase the long term risk of leukaemic transformation. Low dose intermittent oral busulphan may be a convenient alternative in elderly people. Anagrelide is a new agent that can specifically reduce the platelet count and may be useful in conjunction with treatment to control the packed cell volume (see under Essential thrombocythaemia).

Progression—Long survival (>10 years) of the treated patient has revealed a 20% incidence of transformation to myelofibrosis and about 5% to acute leukaemia. The incidence of leukaemia is further increased in those who have transformed to myelofibrosis and those treated with ^{32}P or multiple cytotoxic agents.

Secondary polycythaemia

Many causes of secondary polycythaemia have been identified, the commonest being hypoxaemia (arterial saturation <92%) and renal lesions. In recent years the abuse of drugs such as erythropoietin and anabolic steroids should also be considered in the right context. Investigations are designed to determine the underlying disorder to which the polycythaemia is secondary.

Treatment is aimed at removing the underlying cause when practicable. In hypoxaemia, in which the risk of vascular occlusion is much less pronounced than in polycythaemia vera, venesection is usually undertaken only in those with a very high packed cell volume. At this level the harmful effects of increased viscosity no longer outweigh the oxygen carrying benefits of a raised packed cell volume. Reduction to a packed cell volume of 0.50-0.52 may result in an improvement of cardiopulmonary function. In practice the symptoms experienced by individual patients often decide the target packed cell volume. In polycythaemia associated with renal lesions or other tumours, the packed cell volume should generally be reduced to <0.45.

Apparent polycythaemia

In apparent or relative polycythaemia red cell mass is not increased and the raised packed cell volume is secondary to a decrease in the volume of plasma. An association exists with smoking, alcohol excess, obesity, diuretics, and hypertension.

The need for treatment is uncertain. Lowering the packed cell volume by venesection is undertaken only in patients who have a significantly increased risk of vascular complications for other reasons. On follow up one-third of patients revert spontaneously to a normal packed cell volume.

Box 4.3 Diagnostic criteria for polycythaemia vera

A1 Raised red cell mass
A2 Absence of a cause of secondary polycythaemia
A3 Clinical (palpable) splenomegaly
A4 Bone marrow chromosomal abnormality

B1 Raised neutrophil count ($>10 \times 10^9/l$)
B2 Raised platelet count ($>400 \times 10^9/l$)
B3 Subclinical (radiological) splenomegaly
B4 Erythropoietin-independent erythroid colony (BFU-E) growth or low serum erythropoietin levels

To make the diagnosis of polycythaemia vera:
A1+A2 + A3 or A4, or
A1+A2 + any two of the B criteria

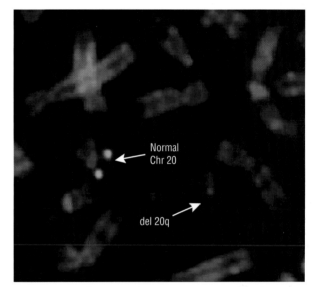

Figure 4.2 Deletion within the long arm of chromosome 20 in polycythaemia vera demonstrated by fluorescent in situ hybridisation. (Red, probe for centromere of chromosome 20; green, probe for long arm of chromosome 20)

Box 4.4 Aims of treatment in polycythaemia vera

• Maintain packed cell volume to <0.45
• Reduce platelet count to $<400 \times 10^9/l$

Box 4.5 Causes of a raised platelet count

• Reactive thrombocytosis
  Infection
  Malignancy
  Inflammatory diseases
  Haemorrhage
  Post-surgery
  Post-splenectomy
• Myeloproliferative disorders
• Chronic myeloid leukaemia
• Myelodysplasia (some forms only)

Essential thrombocythaemia

Like polycythaemia vera and idiopathic myelofibrosis, essential thrombocythaemia is one of the group of clonal conditions known as the myeloproliferative disorders.

A persisting platelet count $>600 \times 10^9$/l is the central diagnostic feature, but other causes of a raised platelet count need to be excluded before a diagnosis of essential thrombocythaemia can be made.

Laboratory investigations

Investigations may reveal other causes of raised platelet count. Apart from a full blood count and blood film they should also include erythrocyte sedimentation rate, serum C reactive protein and serum ferritin, bone marrow aspirate, trephine, and cytogenetic analysis. Although the latter is generally normal in essential thrombocythaemia, certain abnormalities may favour a diagnosis of myelodysplasia or iron deficient (masked) polycythaemia vera and it is important to exclude the presence of a Philadelphia chromosome, which would indicate a diagnosis of chronic myeloid leukaemia.

Presentation and prognosis

Thirty to fifty per cent of patients with essential thrombocythaemia have microvascular occlusive events: for example, burning pain in extremities (erythromelalgia) or digital ischaemia, major vascular occlusive events, or haemorrhage at presentation. These are most pronounced in elderly people, in whom the risk of cerebrovascular accident, myocardial infarction, or other vascular occlusion is high if left untreated. Patients with pre-existing vascular disease will also be at higher risk of such complications. The risk in young patients is lower, though major life threatening events have been described. Transformation to myelofibrosis or acute leukaemia may occur in the long term in a minority of patients.

Treatment and survival

All patients should receive daily low dose aspirin, unless contraindicated because of bleeding or peptic ulceration. This reduces the risk of vascular occlusion but may increase the risk of haemorrhage, particularly at very high platelet counts.

Reduction of the platelet count by cytotoxic agents (daily hydroxyurea, or intermittent low dose busulphan in elderly people) reduces the incidence of vascular complications and appreciably improves survival in older patients (from about three years in untreated patients to 10 years or more in treated patients). The newer drug anagrelide is used increasingly in view of its specificity to the platelet lineage (it selectively inhibits megakaryocyte differentiation) and because of an expectation that it will not increase the long term risk of leukaemic transformation. Interferon α has also been used and is particularly useful in pregnancy.

The Medical Research Council "Primary Thrombocythaemia 1" trial is currently comparing the use of hydroxyurea and anagrelide in patients with essential thrombocythaemia and a high risk of thrombosis.

Idiopathic myelofibrosis

The main features are bone marrow fibrosis, extramedullary haemopoiesis (production of blood cells within organs other than the bone marrow), splenomegaly, and leucoerythroblastic blood picture (immature red and white cells in the peripheral

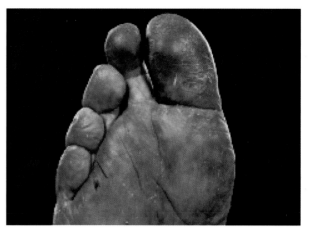

Figure 4.3 Toe ischaemia in a patient with essential thrombocythaemia

Gangrene of the toes in the presence of good peripheral pulses and a raised platelet count strongly suggests primary thrombocythaemia

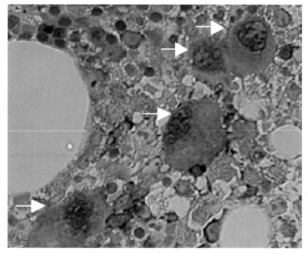

Figure 4.4 Bone marrow trephine biopsy from a patient with essential thrombocythaemia showing clustering of megakaryocytes (arrows)

If there is palpable splenomegaly, a raised platelet count is much more likely to be due to primary thrombocythaemia than to reactive thrombocytosis

The risk of occlusive vascular lesions is very small in reactive thrombocytosis but high in primary thrombocythaemia

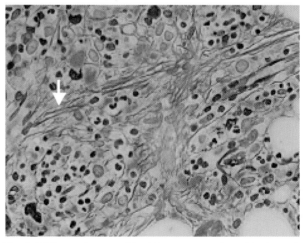

Figure 4.5 Bone marrow trephine biopsy from a patient with advanced idiopathic myelofibrosis. Note the marked linear reticulin staining (arrow)

blood). Good evidence exists that the fibroblast proliferation is secondary (reactive) and not part of the clonal process. In some patients, the fibrosis is accompanied by new bone formation (osteomyelosclerosis). Idiopathic myelofibrosis needs to be distinguished from causes of secondary myelofibrosis (see below).

Presentation
Idiopathic myelofibrosis may have been present for many years before diagnosis. Patients could have had previous undiagnosed primary polycythaemia or thrombocythaemia. The absence of palpable splenomegaly is rare. The main presenting features are abdominal mass (splenomegaly), weight loss (hypermetabolic state), anaemia, fatigue, and bleeding. Fevers and night sweats may be present and are associated with a worse outcome.

Laboratory investigations
A leucoerythroblastic blood picture is characteristic but not diagnostic of idiopathic myelofibrosis as it can occur in cases of marrow infiltration (eg by malignancy, amyloidosis, tuberculosis, osteopetrosis) severe sepsis, severe haemolysis, after administration of haemopoietic growth factors as well as in various types of chronic leukaemia. The blood count is variable. In the initial "proliferative phase" red cell production may be normal or even increased. About half of presenting patients may have a raised white cell count or platelet count (absence of the Philadelphia chromosome will distinguish from chronic myeloid leukaemia). As the bone marrow becomes more fibrotic, the classic "cytopenic phase" supervenes.

Progression and management
The median survival of 2-4 years may be much longer in patients who are asymptomatic at presentation. More recently it has been shown that the presence of anaemia, a very high or low white cell count, the presence of bone marrow chromosomal abnormalities and an advanced patient age are all associated with worse prognosis.

Bone marrow transplantation from a matched sibling or unrelated donor should be offered to young patients with poor prognostic features. This is the only curative treatment modality for myelofibrosis, but in view of its toxicity it cannot be performed in the majority of patients with this disorder, who are over 50 years old at diagnosis.

Supportive blood transfusion may be needed for anaemic patients. Cytotoxic agents may be useful in the proliferative phase, particularly if the platelet count is raised. More recently antifibrotic and antiangiogenic agents such as thalidomide have been used to inhibit progression of fibrosis but success has been limited and there is no convincing evidence that such treatment improves survival. Androgenic steroids such as danazol and oxymethalone can improve the haemoglobin in a proportion of anaemic patients.

Splenectomy may improve the quality of life (though not the prognosis) by reducing the need for transfusions or the pain sometimes associated with a very enlarged spleen. Operative morbidity and mortality can be high and are usually secondary to haemorrhage, making preoperative correction of coagulation abnormalities imperative. Low dose irradiation of the spleen may be helpful in frail patients.

Death can be due to haemorrhage, infection or transformation to acute leukaemia. Portal hypertension with varices, iron overload from blood transfusion, and compression of vital structures by extramedullary haemopoietic masses may also contribute to morbidity.

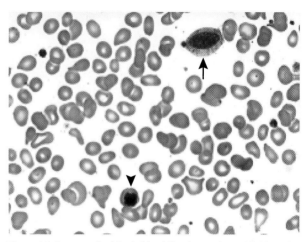

Figure 4.6 Leucoerythroblastic blood film in a patient with idiopathic myelofibrosis. Note the nucleated red blood cell (arrowhead) and the myelocyte (arrow)

Box 4.6 Causes of a leucoerythroblastic blood film

- Idiopathic myelofibrosis
- Bone marrow infiltration
- Severe sepsis
- Severe haemolysis
- Sick neonate

Box 4.7 Bad prognostic features in myelofibrosis

- Hb <10 g/dl
- WCC <4 or >30 × 10^9/l
- Bone marrow chromosomal abnormalities
- Advanced patient age
- Raised number of CD34-positive cells in the peripheral blood

ABC of Clinical Haematology

Further reading
- Bench AJ, Cross CPS, Huntly JP, Nacheva EP, Green AR. Myeloproliferative disorders. Best practice & research. *Clin Haematol* 2001; 3:531-53.
- Pearson TC, Green AR (eds). *Bailliere's clinical haematology.* Myeloproliferative disorders. London: Baillière Tindall, 1998.
- Pearson TC, Messinezy M, Westwood N, *et al.* Polycythemia vera updated: diagnosis, pathobiology, and treatment. *Hemtology* (ASH educational programme book) 2000:51-68.
- Reilly JT. Idiopathic myelofibrosis: pathogenesis, natural history and management. *Blood Rev* 1997; 4:233-42.

We thank Dr Ellie Nacheva for the fluorescent in situ hybridisation image showing deletion of the long arm of chromosome 20 in a bone marrow metaphase from a patient with polycythaemia vera.

5 Chronic myeloid leukaemia

John Goldman

Chronic myeloid leukaemia is a clonal malignant myeloproliferative disorder believed to originate in a single abnormal haemopoietic stem cell. The progeny of this abnormal stem cell proliferate over months or years such that, by the time the leukaemia is diagnosed, the bone marrow is grossly hypercellular and the number of leucocytes is greatly increased in the peripheral blood. Normal blood cell production is almost completely replaced by leukaemia cells, which, however, still function almost normally.

Chronic myeloid leukaemia has an annual incidence of 1 to 1.5 per 100 000 of the population (in the United Kingdom about 700 new cases each year), with no clear geographical variation.

Presentation may be at any age, but the peak incidence is at age 50-70 years, with a slight male predominance. This leukaemia is very rare in children.

Most cases of chronic myeloid leukaemia occur sporadically. The only known predisposing factor is irradiation, as shown by studies of Japanese survivors of the atomic bombs and in patients who received radiotherapy for ankylosing spondylitis.

The clinical course of chronic myeloid leukaemia can be divided into a chronic or "stable" phase and an advanced phase, the latter term covering both accelerated and blastic phases. Most patients present with chronic phase disease, which lasts on average 4-5 years. In about two-thirds of patients the chronic phase transforms gradually into an accelerated phase, characterised by a moderate increase in blast cells, increasing anaemia or thrombocytosis, or other features not compatible with chronic phase disease. After a variable number of months this accelerated phase progresses to frank acute blastic transformation. The remaining one-third of patients move abruptly from chronic phase to an acute blastic phase (or blastic crisis) without an intervening phase of acceleration.

Pathogenesis

All leukaemia cells in patients with chronic myeloid leukaemia contain a specific cytogenetic marker, described originally in 1960 by workers in Philadelphia and now known as the Philadelphia or Ph chromosome.

The Ph chromosome is derived from a normal 22 chromosome that has lost part of its long arm as a result of a balanced reciprocal translocation of chromosomal material involving one of the 22 and one of the 9 chromosomes. The translocation is usually referred to as t(9;22)(q34;q11). Thus the Ph chromosome (also known as 22q−) appears somewhat shorter than its normal counterpart and the 9q+ somewhat longer than the normal 9.

The Ph chromosome carries a specific fusion gene known as BCR-ABL, which results from juxtaposition with part of the ABL proto-oncogene (from chromosome 9) with part of the BCR gene on chromosome 22. This fusion gene is expressed as a specific messenger RNA (mRNA), which in turn generates a protein called p210$^{BCR-ABL}$. This protein perturbs stem cell kinetics, resulting in the chronic phase of chronic myeloid leukaemia, although the exact mechanism remains unclear.

Researchers have recently developed a drug (imatinib mesylate) that blocks the action of the BCR-ABL gene and thereby reverses the leukaemic phenotype in chronic myeloid leukaemia cells.

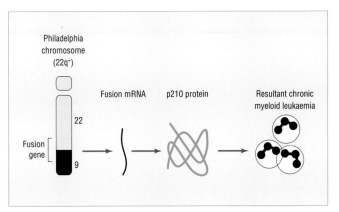

Figure 5.1 Formation of the Philadelphia chromosome resulting in a BCR-ABL fusion gene that generates a fusion protein (p210) responsible for the chronic myeloid leukaemia phenotype

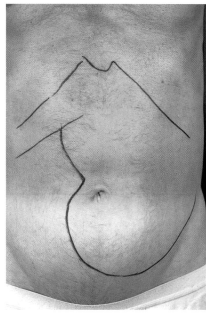

Figure 5.2 Patient with massive splenomegaly in chronic phase chronic myeloid leukaemia

Box 5.3 Usual peripheral blood findings in chronic myeloid leukaemia at diagnosis
- Raised white blood cell count ($30\text{-}400 \times 10^9$/l).
  Differential shows:
    Granulocytes at all stages of development
    Increased numbers of basophils and eosinophils
    Blast (primitive) cells (maximum 10%)—never present in the blood of normal people
- Haemoglobin concentration may be reduced; red cell morphology is usually unremarkable; nucleated (immature) red cells may be present
- Platelet count may be raised ($300\text{-}600 \times 10^9$/l)

The spleen may be greatly enlarged before onset of symptoms. Treatment that reduces leucocyte count to normal usually restores the spleen to normal size

Chronic phase disease

Presentation

The characteristic symptoms at presentation include fatigue, weight loss, sweating, anaemia, haemorrhage or purpura, and the sensation of a mass in the left upper abdominal quadrant (spleen). Often the disease is detected as a result of routine blood tests performed for unrelated reasons, and a fifth of patients are totally asymptomatic at the time of diagnosis. The spleen may be greatly enlarged before onset of symptoms. Treatment that reduces the leucocyte count to normal usually restores the spleen to normal size. Much rarer features at presentation include non-specific fever, lymphadenopathy, visual disturbances due to leucostasis (a form of hyperviscosity caused by an extremely high white cell count) or retinal haemorrhages, splenic pain due to infarction, gout, and occasionally priapism.

The commonest physical sign at diagnosis is an enlarged spleen, which may vary from being just palpable at the left costal margin to filling the whole left side of the abdomen and extending towards the right iliac fossa. The liver may be enlarged, with a soft, rather ill defined lower edge. Spontaneous and excessive bruising in response to minor trauma is common.

Diagnosis

The diagnosis of chronic myeloid leukaemia in chronic phase can be made from study of the peripheral blood film, which shows greatly increased numbers of leucocytes with many immature forms (promyelocytes and myelocytes); the marrow is usually examined to confirm the diagnosis.

Marrow examination shows increased cellularity. The distribution of immature leucocytes resembles that seen in the blood film. Red cell production is relatively reduced. Megakaryocytes, the cells giving rise to platelets, are plentiful but may be smaller than usual.

Cytogenetic study of marrow shows the presence of the Ph chromosome in all dividing cells.

The patient's blood concentrations of urea and electrolytes are usually normal at diagnosis, whereas the lactate dehydrogenase is usually raised. Serum urate concentration may be raised.

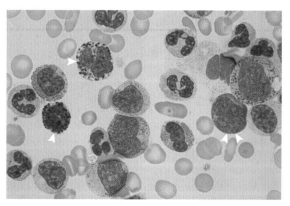

Figure 5.3 Peripheral blood film from patient with chronic myeloid leukaemia showing many mature granulocytes, including two basophils (arrow); a blast cell is prominent (double arrow)

Box 5.4 Investigations to confirm suspected chronic myeloid leukaemia

Routine
- Full blood count including blood film
- Neutrophil alkaline phosphatase
- Urea, electrolytes
- Serum lactate dehydrogenase
- Bone marrow aspirate (degree of cellularity, chromosome analysis)

Optional
- Bone marrow trephine biopsy (extent of fibrosis)
- BCR-ABL chimeric gene by fluorescent in situ hybridisation or by polymerase chain reaction
- Vitamin B_{12} and B_{12} binding capacity
- HLA typing for patient and family members

Management

After diagnosis, the first priority is a frank discussion with the patient. It is now customary to use the term leukaemia in this discussion and to explain to the patient that he or she may expect to live for several years with a near normal lifestyle. The clinician should explain the propensity of the disease to progress to an advanced phase. The choice of treatment with imatinib mesylate (STI571, Glivec), interferon α or hydroxyurea should be discussed.

If chronic myeloid leukaemia is diagnosed in pregnancy the woman should have the chance to continue to term. Chronic myeloid leukaemia has no adverse effect on pregnancy and pregnancy has no adverse effect on the leukaemia.

The clinician may wish to mention at this point the existence of patient information booklets produced by BACUP (British Association of Cancer United Patients) and by the Leukaemia Research Fund, which are extremely valuable as many patients will not retain all that is said at this first interview. There are also a number of useful websites available on the Internet, though some of these are somewhat one-sided.

Imatinib mesylate (STI571)—Imatinib mesylate has just become generally available and seems already to be the treatment of choice for chronic myeloid leukaemia presenting in chronic phase. It acts by specifically inhibiting the enhanced protein tyrosine kinase activity of the BCR-ABL oncoprotein and thus reversing the pathologically perturbed signal transduction. Preliminary clinical studies show that it induces complete haematological remission in >95% of previously untreated patients and at least 50% of these will achieve a complete cytogenetic remission. Toxicity seems to be relatively mild. It is too early to say whether the drug will prolong life in comparison with interferon α used alone or in conjunction with cytarabine.

Interferon α—Interferon α is a member of a family of naturally occurring glycoproteins with antiviral and antiproliferative actions. It was until recently the drug of choice for managing chronic myeloid leukaemia in the chronic phase. It restores spleen size and blood counts to normal in 70-80% of patients. Some 10-20% of patients achieve a major reduction or complete disappearance of cells with the Ph chromosome from their bone marrow (tantamount to complete cytogenetic remission). Interferon α initially causes flu-like symptoms, but these usually subside. Other more persistent side effects include anorexia, weight loss, depression, alopecia, rashes, neuropathies, autoimmune disorders, and thrombocytopenia. Currently interferon α should be considered for chronic phase patients resistant to imatinib mesylate.

Allogeneic stem cell transplantation—Patients under the age of 60 years who have siblings with identical HLA types may be offered treatment by high dose cytoreduction (chemotherapy and radiotherapy) followed by transplantation of haemopoietic stem cells collected from the donor's bone marrow or peripheral blood. With typical family size in western Europe, about 30% of patients will have matched sibling donors. In selected cases transplants may also be performed with HLA-identical unrelated donors. Allogeneic stem cell transplants are associated with an appreciable risk of morbidity and mortality, and in general, older patients (aged 40-60) fare less well than younger patients. Nevertheless, the projected cure rate after allogeneic stem cell transplantation is about 60-70%.

Autologous stem cell transplantation—For patients up to the age of 65 years for whom an allograft is excluded, autografting may be considered. For this purpose haemopoietic stem cells are collected from the patient's blood or marrow and cryopreserved. The patient then receives high dose

Box 5.5 Treatment with hydroxyurea

- Hydroxyurea inhibits the enzyme ribonucleotide reductase and acts specifically on cells of the myeloid series—ie neutrophils, eosinophils, basophils, etc
- It is useful for rapid reduction of the leucocyte count in newly diagnosed patients
- Many haematologists start treatment with hydroxyurea then switch to interferon α once the patient's symptoms are relieved and the leucocyte count is restored to normal
- Hydroxyurea is also valuable for controlling chronic phase disease in patients who cannot tolerate interferon α
- It is usually started at 2.0 g daily by mouth; the usual maintenance dose is 1.0-1.5 g daily, titrated against the leucocyte count
- Treatment with hydroxyurea does not eradicate cells with the Ph chromosome
- Side effects are rare but include rashes, mouth ulceration, and gastrointestinal symptoms. The drug causes macrocytosis and megaloblastoid changes in the marrow

Younger men should be offered cryopreservation of semen if necessary

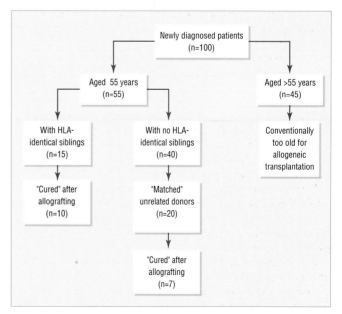

Figure 5.4 Eligibility for and results of allogeneic transplantation for unselected 100 newly diagnosed patients

cytoreductive chemotherapy, followed by reinfusion of the thawed stem cells. The procedure may prolong life in some cases, and remains experimental.

Advanced phase disease

Presentation
Advanced phase disease may be diagnosed incidentally as a result of a blood test at a routine clinic visit. Alternatively the patient may have excessive sweating, persistent fever, or otherwise unexplained symptoms of anaemia, splenic enlargement or splenic infarction, haemorrhage, or bone pain. In most cases the blast crisis is myeloid (that is, resembling acute myeloid leukaemia), and in a fifth of cases lymphoid blast crisis occurs.

Occasionally patients progress to a myelofibrotic phase of the disease, in which intense marrow fibrosis predominates, blast cells proliferate less aggressively, and the clinical picture is characterised by splenomegaly and pancytopenia consequent on marrow failure.

Management
Patients in accelerated phase may derive considerable benefit from imatinib mesylate, which can re-establish chronic phase disease and even Ph-negative haemopoiesis in some cases. They may also respond to hydroxyurea or busulphan if they have not previously received these agents. Splenectomy may be useful to improve thrombocytopenia or symptoms due to splenomegaly. Patients in a blastic phase respond only transiently to imatinib mesylate. It is probably preferable to rely on the use of combination chemotherapy, though the possibility of treating localised pain or resistant splenomegaly by radiotherapy should not be forgotten. For those patients with myeloid transformations, drugs suitable for treating acute myeloid leukaemia will control the leukaemic proliferation for a time. About 30% of patients will achieve a second chronic phase compatible with a normal lifestyle for months or years. Patients with lymphoid transformations should be treated with drugs appropriate to adult acute lymphoblastic leukaemia. Second chronic phase may be achieved in 40-60% of cases, more commonly in those who had a short interval from diagnosis to transformation. Patients restored to second chronic phase should receive prophylaxis against neuroleukaemia, comprising five or six intrathecal injections of methotrexate, but there is no indication for cranial or craniospinal irradiation.

Box 5.6 Criteria for advanced phase disease

- Increasing splenomegaly despite full doses of cytotoxic drugs
- Rapid white blood cell doubling time
- White blood cell count poorly responsive to full doses of cytotoxic drugs
- Anaemia or thrombocytopenia unresponsive to cytotoxic drugs
- Persistent thrombocytosis ($>1000 \times 10^9/l$)
- >10% blasts in peripheral blood or marrow
- >20% blasts plus promyelocytes in blood or marrow
- Acquisition of "non-random" chromosomal changes in addition to presence of Philadelphia chromosome
- Development of myelofibrosis

At times the advanced phase can be difficult to distinguish from the chronic phase and can be diagnosed with confidence only in retrospect

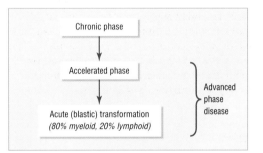

Figure 5.5 Progression of chronic myeloid leukaemia, showing progression to blastic phase

---

Further reading

- Sawyers C. Chronic myeloid leukemia. *N Engl J Med* 1999;340: 1330-40.
- Deininger M, Goldman JM, Melo JM. The molecular biology of chronic myeloid leukemia. *Blood* 2000;96:3343-56.
- Hasford J, Pfirrmann J, Hehlmann R *et al.* A new prognostic score for survival of patients with chronic myeloid leukemia treated with interferon alfa. *JNCI* 1998;90:850-8.
- Guilhot F, Chastang C, Michallet M *et al.* Interferon alpha 2b combined with cytarabine versus interferon alone in chronic myelogenous leukemia. *N Engl J Med* 1997;337:223-9.
- Goldman JM, Druker B. Chronic myeloid leukemia: current treatment options. *Blood* 2001;98:2039-42.
- Kantarjian H, Sawyers C, Hochhaus A *et al.* Hematologic and cytogenetic responses to imatinib mesylate in chronic myelogenous leukemia. *N Engl J Med* 2002;346;645-52.

6 The acute leukaemias

T Everington, R J Liesner, A H Goldstone

Acute leukaemia is a clonal (that is, derived from a single cell) malignant disorder affecting all age groups with an average annual incidence rate of 4-7 people per 100 000. It is characterised by the accumulation of immature blast cells in the bone marrow, which replace normal marrow tissue, including haemopoietic precursor cells. This results in bone marrow failure, reflected by peripheral blood cytopenias and circulating blast cells. Infiltration of various organs is also a feature of some forms of leukaemia.

In most cases the aetiology is not obvious, but internal and external factors associated with damage to DNA can predispose to acute leukaemia. Over 50 years, progressive advances in the treatment of acute leukaemia have converted an incurable disease to one in which complete remissions can be obtained in up to 95% of selected patients treated with curative intent. This has largely been the result of ongoing clinical trials, improved supportive treatment and the development of bone marrow transplantation for those in higher risk categories.

Classification

Acute leukaemia is subdivided into (a) acute lymphoblastic leukaemia (ALL), in which the abnormal proliferation is in the lymphoid progenitor cells (that is, immature lymphocytes) and (b) acute myeloid leukaemia (AML), which involves the myeloid lineages (that is, cells from which neutrophils, eosinophils, monocytes, basophils, megakaryocytes, etc. are derived). The distinction between the two leukaemias is based on morphological, cytochemical, immunological and cytogenetic differences and is of paramount importance as the treatment and prognosis are usually different.

Both acute lymphoblastic leukaemia and acute myeloid leukaemia are currently further subdivided on the basis of morphological criteria: acute lymphoblastic leukaemia into FAB (French-American-British) subtypes L1, L2, and L3, and acute myeloid leukaemia into FAB subtypes M0 to M7.

On the basis of surface antigen expression, acute lymphoblastic leukaemia is divided into T cell lineage and B cell lineage. B cell lineage is further subdivided: early B precursor acute lymphoblastic leukaemia is the most immature and is negative for the common acute lymphoblastic leukaemia antigen (CD 10); common acute lymphoblastic leukaemia and pre-B cell acute lymphoblastic leukaemia are more mature and are CD 10 positive; and B cell acute lymphoblastic leukaemia is the most mature and is the only one to express surface immunoglobulin. Little correlation exists between morphological subtype and immunophenotype or prognosis in L1 or L2 acute lymphoblastic leukaemia. L3 morphology is almost exclusively found in B cell acute lymphoblastic leukaemia.

In acute myeloid leukaemia immunophenotyping may not help to distinguish between leukaemias of the myeloid (M0 to M3), the myelomonocytic (M4), and the monocytic (M5) lineages, and special cytochemical stains are usually used to support morphological findings. In erythroleukaemia (M6) and megakaryoblastic leukaemia (M7), however, the surface antigen expression is often diagnostic.

The FAB classification system, while essentially simple, has several deficiencies, not least a lack of clear

Box 6.1 Aetiological factors in acute leukaemia

- Unknown (usually)
- Hereditary
  Down's syndrome
  Bloom's syndrome
  Fanconi's anaemia
  Ataxia telangiectasia
  Kleinfelter's syndrome
  Osteogenesis imperfecta
  Wiskott-Aldrich syndrome
  Leukaemia in siblings
- Chemicals
  Chronic benzene exposure
  Alkylating agents (chlorambucil, melphalan)
- Radiation
- Predisposing haematological diseases (myeloproliferative disorders, myelodysplasia, and aplastic anaemia)
- Viruses (HTLV-I causing adult T cell leukaemia/lymphoma)

Box 6.2 FAB* Classification of acute myeloid leukaemia

M0	Acute myeloid leukaemia with minimal evidence of myeloid differentiation
M1	Acute myeloblastic leukaemia without maturation
M2	Acute myeloblastic leukaemia with maturation
M3	Acute promyelocytic leukaemia
M4	Acute myelomonocytic leukaemia
M5	Acute monocytic/monoblastic leukaemia
M6	Acute erythroleukaemia
M7	Acute megakaryoblastic leukaemia

*French-American-British

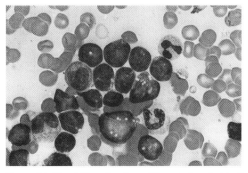

Figure 6.1 Blood film of patient with acute lymphoblastic leukaemia

diagnostic/prognostic association. A Clinical Advisory Committee to the World Health Organization (WHO) has now published a new classification system which is based around cytogenetic abnormalities, and which thereby seeks to define biological and clinical entities more closely. It is likely that this will be adopted in the near future.

Incidence

Acute lymphoblastic leukaemia

Acute lymphoblastic leukaemia is most common in the age range 2-10 years, with a peak at 3-4 years. The incidence then decreases with increasing age, though there is a secondary rise after 40 years. In children it is the most common malignant disease and accounts for 85% of childhood leukaemia.

Acute myeloid leukaemia

Acute myeloid leukaemia accounts for 10-15% of childhood leukaemia, but it is the commonest leukaemia of adulthood, particularly as chronic myeloproliferative disorders and preleukaemic conditions such as myelodysplasia usually progress to acute myeloid leukaemia rather than acute lymphoblastic leukaemia. The incidence increases with age, and the median age at presentation is 60 years.

Presentation

Acute leukaemia is always serious and life threatening, and all patients suspected of having this condition should be immediately referred for urgent assessment.

Common symptoms and signs at presentation result from bone marrow failure or, less commonly, organ infiltration. Anaemia can result in pallor, lethargy, and dyspnoea. Neutropenia results in predominantly bacterial infections of the mouth, throat, skin, chest or perianal region. Thrombocytopenia may present as spontaneous bruising, menorrhagia, bleeding from venepuncture sites, gingival bleeding, or prolonged nose bleeds.

A common presenting feature resulting from organ infiltration in childhood acute lymphoblastic leukaemia is bone pain, but acute lymphoblastic leukaemia can also present with superficial lymphadenopathy, abdominal distension due to abdominal lymphadenopathy and hepatosplenomegaly, respiratory embarrassment due to a large mediastinal mass, testicular enlargement, or a meningeal syndrome. Gum hypertrophy and skin infiltration are more commonly seen in acute myeloid than in acute lymphoblastic leukaemia.

Investigations

Full blood count usually but not invariably shows reduced haemoglobin concentration and platelet count. The white cell count can vary from $<1.0 \times 10^9/l$ to $>200 \times 10^9/l$, and the differential white cell count is often abnormal, with neutropenia and the presence of blast cells. The anaemia is a normochromic, normocytic anaemia, and the thrombocytopenia may be severe (platelet count $<10 \times 10^9/l$).

Coagulation screening may yield abnormal results, particularly in promyelocytic leukaemia (acute myeloid leukaemia M3) when granules from the leukaemic blasts can have procoagulant activity and trigger a consumptive coagulopathy.

Biochemical screening is particularly important if the leucocyte count is very high, when there may be evidence of renal impairment and hyperuricaemia.

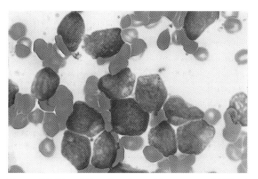

Figure 6.2 Blood film of patient with acute myeloid leukaemia

> **Acute lymphoblastic leukaemia is slightly more common among males than females**

> **Acute myeloid leukaemia is equally common among males and females**

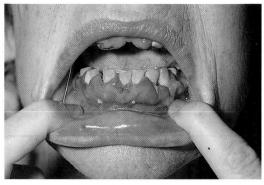

Figure 6.3 Severe gum swelling at presentation in acute myeloid leukaemia M5

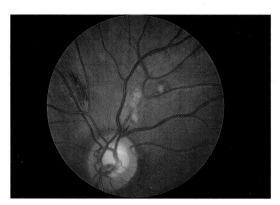

Figure 6.4 Infiltration of optic fundus by acute lymphoblastic leukaemia

Box 6.3 Differential diagnosis of acute leukaemia

- If lymphadenopathy: infections such as infectious mononucleosis or lymphoma
- If hepatosplenomegaly: myeloproliferative or lymphoproliferative disorder, myelodysplasia, metabolic, storage or autoimmune disorders (rarely, tropical disease, eg visceral leishmaniasis)
- If no peripheral leukaemic blasts but pancytopenia: aplastic anaemia or infiltrated bone marrow involvement from non-haemopoietic small round cell tumour
- Myelodysplasia
- Lymphoblastic lymphoma: lymphomatous presentation with <25% of blasts in the marrow (distinction may be arbitrary as treatment may be the same)

Chest radiography is mandatory to exclude the presence of a mediastinal mass, which is present in up to 70% of patients with T cell acute lymphoblastic leukaemia. In childhood acute lymphoblastic leukaemia lytic bone lesions may also be seen.

Bone marrow aspiration with or without trephination is essential to confirm acute leukaemia. The marrow is usually hypercellular, with a predominance of immature (blast) cells.

Immunophenotyping of the antigens present on blasts isolated from the bone marrow or peripheral blood is the most reliable method of determining whether the leukaemia is lymphoid or myeloid, and cytochemistry helps to confirm myeloid or monocytic origin.

Cytogenetics and molecular studies often detect abnormalities within the leukaemic clone that can have diagnostic or prognostic value—for example, the Philadelphia chromosome, which is the product of a translocation between chromosomes 9 and 22, the presence of which confers a very poor prognosis in cases of acute lymphoblastic leukaemia.

Atraumatic lumbar puncture with cerebrospinal fluid cytospin is an important initial staging investigation in ALL or AML with neurological symptoms to detect leukaemic cells in the cerebrospinal fluid, indicating involvement of the central nervous system.

Management

All patients who have either suspected or confirmed acute leukaemia should be referred for specialist advice, assessment, and treatment. Which centre a patient is referred to, and the type of treatment given, will depend on the patient's age and condition. Children and young adults should always be treated in recognized specialist centres to maximise the chance of cure with minimal toxicity. On admission to a specialist unit the patient will need chemotherapy to treat the leukaemia and supportive care to ameliorate or correct the effects of the leukaemia and to facilitate treatment.

Supportive care

The numerical threshold for blood product transfusion has progressively lowered. Prophylactic platelet transfusions are given if the platelet count is $<10 \times 10^9/l$. Bleeding episodes predominantly result from thrombocytopenia and should be treated accordingly. Clotting abnormalities may result from a consumptive coagulopathy where infusions of fresh frozen plasma and cryoprecipitate may be beneficial. Packed red cell transfusions are given for symptomatic anaemia, though these are contraindicated if the white cell count is extremely high.

In most patients a central venous catheter has to be inserted to facilitate blood product support, administration of chemotherapy and antibiotics, and frequent blood sampling.

Serious infection is a common cause of death in patients with acute leukaemia, as bone marrow failure due to the leukaemia and to chemotherapy often results in profound neutropenia for two weeks or more. Reverse-barrier nursing techniques should therefore be used for such patients, and intravenous antimicrobial agents should be started as soon as there is a fever or other sign of infection.

Chemotherapy

The aim of chemotherapy for leukaemia is initially to induce a remission (<5% blasts in the bone marrow) and then to eradicate the residual leukaemic cell population by further courses of consolidation therapy. The drugs damage the capacity of the leukaemic cells to divide and replicate, and using cyclical combinations of three or more drugs increases

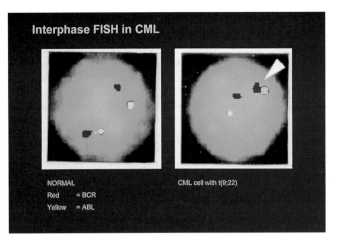

Figure 6.5 Interphase fluorescent in situ hybridisation using probes for BCR and ABL genes. Left: Normal cell showing two red dots (two normal copies of BCR) and two yellow dots (two normal copies of ABL). Right: Cell from child with Ph chromosome positive acute lymphoblastic leukaemia with translocation of chromosomes 9 and 22

Box 6.4 Management of acute leukaemia

- Immediate (same day) referral to specialist
- Prompt diagnosis
- Early treatment
- Intensive supportive care
- Systemic chemotherapy
- Treatment directed at central nervous system (in children and in adult acute lymphoblastic leukaemia)
- Minimising early and late toxicity of treatment

Adequate hydration and allopurinol are essential at the start of treatment to reduce the risk of hyperkalaemia, hyperuricaemia, and renal damage

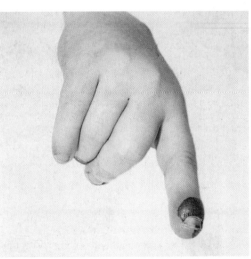

Figure 6.6 Pseudomonas infection of skin and nail bed in patient having treatment for acute myeloid leukaemia

Psychological and social support to patients and families of patients with leukaemia is important, and specialist centres have networks to provide this

the cytotoxic effect, improves the chance of remission after the initial "induction" period, and reduces the emergence of drug resistance. In Britain acute myeloid leukaemia is currently treated with four or five courses of intensive chemotherapy when there is intent to cure. Each course entails up to 10 days of chemotherapy. Subsequent courses are commenced after cell counts have recovered and response to treatment is established. During the recovery phase the patient is severely myelosuppressed and needs inpatient blood product support and antimicrobial drugs. In acute myeloid leukaemia M3 the drug ATRA (all-trans-retinoic acid) is used as an adjunct to chemotherapy as it causes differentiation of the malignant clone.

In acute lymphoblastic leukaemia the induction course is followed by two or more consolidation periods and by treatment directed at the central nervous system (see below), followed by long term maintenance or continuation treatment for up to two years. This has been shown to improve long term cure rates in acute lymphoblastic leukaemia, though not in acute myeloid leukaemia.

Some aggressive leukaemia subtypes such as adult T cell leukaemia and Burkitt's lymphoma/leukaemia have shown marked responsiveness to short term intensive treatment schedules. Complete remission rates of 65-86% have been achieved in a disease that previously had an extremely poor prognosis.

Treatment directed at the central nervous system

The treatment or prevention of leukaemic cells in the central nervous system is part of all treatment protocols in childhood leukaemia and adult acute lymphoblastic leukaemia, but not in adults with acute myeloid leukaemia unless they have symptoms or blasts are present in the cerebrospinal fluid. Treatment directed at the central nervous system generally comprises regular intrathecal chemotherapy (usually methotrexate), high dose intravenous methotrexate, or cranial irradiation.

Bone marrow transplantation

Up to 85% of patients who initially achieve a complete remission will subsequently relapse. Transplantation reduces relapse risk but has been associated with high procedural mortality. The development of peripheral rather than bone marrow stem cell harvest has reduced procedural mortality.

The principle of dose intensity suggests that higher doses of chemotherapy will reduce relapse risk. Autologous transplantation involves stem cell rescue (with patients' own cells harvested in remission) after a potentially lethal dose of chemotherapy. Ongoing large scale clinical trials are studying the benefit of this modality over conventional treatment.

The concept of allogeneic transplantation—where healthy stem cells from a sibling or unrelated donor are given to replace diseased marrow—has always been appealing. Realisation of a graft versus leukaemia (GVL) effect has enhanced enthusiasm, though this effect is more pronounced in chronic myeloid leukaemia. "Mini" allografts exploit GVL; non-myeloablative doses of chemotherapy induce a state of marrow chimaerism where persistent minimal residual disease may be eradicated by donor lymphocyte infusion.

Patient selection for BMT remains a subject of controversy. Some patients will self-exclude on personal, age or health grounds. Others may be suitable for BMT but not have an appropriate donor. This problem is likely to worsen as family size reduces and volunteer healthy donors are harder to attract.

Table 6.1 Poor prognosis in acute lymphoblastic leukaemia

Factors	Acute lymphoblastic leukaemia
Age	<1 year or >10 years
Sex	Male
Presenting white blood cells	>50 × 10^9/l
Central nervous system disease	Presence of blasts in cerebrospinal fluid at presentation
Remission problems	Failure to remit after first induction treatment
Cytogenetics	Philadelphia positive—that is, t(9;22)—or t(4;11)acute lymphoblastic leukaemia

Table 6.2 Poor prognosis in acute myeloid leukaemia

Factors	Acute myeloid leukaemia
Age	>60 years
Sex	Male or female
Presenting white blood cells	>50 × 10^9/l
Central nervous system disease	Presence of blasts in cerebrospinal fluid at presentation (rare)
Remission problems	>20% blasts in bone marrow after first course of treatment
Cytogenetics	Deletions or monosomy of chromosome 5 or 7 or complex chromosomal abnormalities

Box 6.5 Ongoing Medical Research Council clinical trials

- Acute lymphoblastic leukaemia in both children and adults
- Relapsed acute lymphoblastic leukaemia in children
- Acute myeloid leukaemia in patients aged <60 years
- Acute myeloid leukaemia in patients aged >55 years

Table 6.3 Survival with acute leukaemia

Type	At 5 years
Childhood acute lymphoblastic leukaemia	65-75%
Adult acute lymphoblastic leukaemia	20-45%
Acute myeloid leukaemia, aged <60 years	35-40%
Acute myeloid leukaemia, aged >60 years	10%

Novel developments

The majority of new presentations with acute leukaemia occur in the older population. Whilst complete remission may be obtained with standard treatment in up to 62% of this group, only 8-12% will be alive at five years. This phenomenon is due to the increased finding of adverse karyotype, chemoresistant phenotype, and disease evolution from myelodysplastic syndrome together with comorbidity and poor tolerance of chemotherapy in this population. This, together with the knowledge that patients who relapse have three year survival rates of 8%, has driven the search for alternative but potentially synergistic modalities of treatment.

Gemtuzumab ozogamicin (GO) is a humanised monoclonal antibody to CD33, an antigen found on >80% of blasts in AML, conjugated to the anti-tumour antibiotic calicheamicin. Patients treated in first relapse AML show 30% complete remission with single agent GO and reasonable toxicity profiles. This agent is being incorporated into the latest AML studies.

STI 571 is a tyrosine kinase (TK) inhibitor which has good activity in chronic myeloid leukaemia due to the presence of the Philadelphia chromosome associated with aberrant TK production. The Philadelphia chromosome is found in 20-30% adult ALL and is associated with extremely poor prognosis. STI may be of benefit in this group and also in those with AML who show Flt 3 mutations, also associated with aberrant TK.

The multi-drug resistant genotype (MDR) results in patients phenotypically showing resistance to a spectrum of drugs by causing them to efflux from cells before exerting their cytotoxic effect. Inhibitory drugs to this process are in advanced stages of development. A few of the many other fields of development showing potential are anti-angiogenic drugs, anti-leukaemic vaccines and tumour-specific cytotoxic T cell therapy. It is increasingly understood that acute leukaemia is a highly heterogeneous condition which requires an individualised approach to management.

Toxicity of therapy

Early side effects

Most chemotherapeutic agents have pronounced side effects, such as nausea and vomiting, mucositis, hair loss, neuropathy, and renal and hepatic dysfunction. Many also cause myelosuppression, resulting in profound neutropenia for two or more weeks with resultant opportunistic infection. Febrile neutropenic episodes require prompt use of broad spectrum antibiotics. Many patients also develop fungal infection requiring treatment with systemic antifungal drugs. Viral infection is predominantly seen in the post-transplant setting.

Late effects

All treatments for acute leukaemia can result in long term side effects that may bring appreciable morbidity or even lead to death. Patients must therefore be followed up in a specialist unit for at least 10 years. Particular attention must be paid to the long term problems with growth and endocrine function in children.

Box 6.6 Late effects of treatment for acute leukaemia

- **Cardiac:** Arrhythmias, cardiomyopathy
- **Pulmonary:** Fibrosis
- **Endocrine:** Growth delay, hypothyroidism, gonadal dysfunction or failure, infertility
- **Renal:** Reduced glomerular filtration rate
- **Psychological:** Intellectual dysfunction, long term anxiety about relapse
- **Second malignancy:** Secondary leukaemias or solid tumours
- **Cataracts**

Further reading

- Burnett A. Acute myeloid leukaemia *Clin Haematol* 2001;14(1).
- Kantarjian H, Hoelzer D, Larson R. Advances in the treatment of acute lymphocytic leukaemia *Hematol/Oncol Clin North Am* 2000;14(6) and 2001;15(1).
- Gorin N. New developments in the therapy of acute myelocytic leukaemia. *Am Soc Hematol Educ Progr* 2000;69-89.
- Appelbaum F, Rowe J, Radich J, Dick J. Acute myeloid leukaemia. *Am Soc Hematol Educ Progr* 2001;62-86.
- Hoelzer D, Burnett A. Acute leukaemias in adults. In *Oxford textbook of oncology*, 2nd edn. Oxford: Oxford University Press, 2002;2191-2212.
- Grimwade D, Walker H, Oliver F *et al.* on behalf of the Medical Research Council Adult and Children's Leukaemia Working Parties. The importance of diagnostic cytogenetics on outcome in AML: Analysis of 1,612 patients entered into the MRC AML10 trial *Blood* 1998;92(7):2322-33.
- Goldstone A, Burnett A, Wheatley K, Smith A, Hutchinson RM, Clark RE on behalf of the Medical Research Council Adult Leukaemia Working Party. Attempts to improve treatment outcomes in AML in older patients: The results of the UK MRC AML11 trial. *Blood* 2001;98(5):1302-11.
- Yin J, Wheatley K, Rees J, Burnett A on behalf of the UK MRC Adult Leukaemia Working Party. Comparison of 'sequential' versus 'standard' chemotherapy as re-induction treatment, with or without cyclosporine, in refractory/relapsed AML: results of the UK MRC AML-R trial. *Br J Haematol* 2001;113:713-26.
- Sievers E, Larson R, Stadtmauer E *et al.* for the Mylotarg Study Group. Efficacy and safety of Mylotarg (gemtuzumab ozogamicin) in patients with CD33-positive acute myeloid leukemia in first relapse. *J Clin Oncol* (in press).

The interphase fluorescent in situ hybridisation was provided by Brian Reeves and Helen Kempski, Department of Haematology, Great Ormond Street Hospital for Children NHS Trust, London.

7 Platelet disorders

R J Liesner, S J Machin

Platelets are produced predominantly by the bone marrow megakaryocytes as a result of budding of the cytoplasmic membrane. Megakaryocytes are derived from the haemopoetic stem cell, which is stimulated to differentiate to mature megakaryocytes under the influence of various cytokines, including thrombopoietin. Once released from the bone marrow young platelets are trapped in the spleen for up to 36 hours before entering the circulation, where they have a primary haemostatic role. Their normal lifespan is 7-10 days and the normal platelet count for all age groups is $150\text{-}450 \times 10^9/\text{l}$. The mean platelet diameter is 1-2 μm and the normal range for cell volume (MPV) is 8-11 fl. Although platelets are non-nucleated cells, those that have recently been released from the bone marrow contain RNA and are known as reticulated platelets. They normally represent 8-16% of the total count and they indirectly indicate the state of marrow production.

Normal haemostasis

The platelet membrane has integral glycoproteins essential in the initial events of adhesion and aggregation, leading to formation of the platelet plug during haemostasis.

Glycoprotein receptors react with aggregating agents such as collagen on the damaged vascular endothelial surface, fibrinogen, and von Willebrand factor to facilitate platelet-platelet and platelet-endothelial cell adhesion. The major glycoproteins are the Ib-IX complex, whose main binding protein is von Willebrand factor, and IIb/IIIa which specifically binds fibrinogen. Storage organelles within the platelet include the "dense" granules which contain nucleotides, calcium and serotonin, and α granules containing fibrinogen, von Willebrand factor, platelet-derived growth factor and many other clotting factors. Following adhesion, the platelets are stimulated to release the contents of their granules essential for platelet aggregation. The platelets also provide an extensive phospholipid surface for the interaction and activation of clotting factors in the coagulation pathway.

Congenital abnormalities

Congenital abnormalities of platelets can be divided into disorders of platelet production and those of platelet function. All are very rare. In general they cause moderate to severe bleeding problems.

Fanconi's anaemia is an autosomal recessive preleukaemic condition which often presents as thrombocytopenia with skeletal or genitourinary abnormalities. The cardinal laboratory feature is abnormal chromosomal fragility. The condition can be cured with bone marrow transplantation (BMT).

Thrombocytopenia with absent radii (TAR syndrome) presents with the pathognomic sign of bilateral absent radii and with severe ($<10 \times 10^9/\text{l}$) neonatal thrombocytopenia, though this often improves after the first year of life. This should be distinguished from *amegakaryocytic thrombocytopenia*, another leukaemia predisposition syndrome, in which severe neonatal thrombocytopenia is present with or without somatic abnormalities.

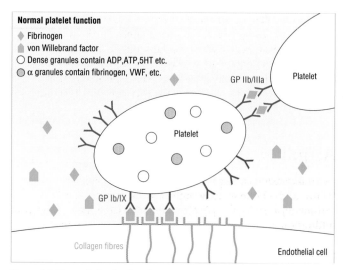

Figure 7.1 Normal platelet function

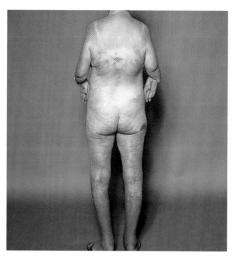

Figure 7.2 Amegakaryocytic thrombocytopenia with absent radii (TAR syndrome)

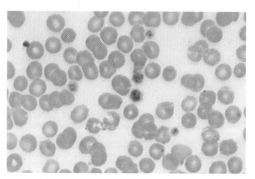

Figure 7.3 Giant granular platelets in peripheral blood film as seen in Bernard-Soulier syndrome or May Hegglin anomaly

The Wiskott-Aldrich syndrome is an X-linked disorder with a triad of thrombocytopenia, eczema, and immunodeficiency. The platelet count is usually $20\text{-}100 \times 10^9/l$, and the platelets are small and functionally abnormal. Like Fanconi's anaemia, this condition can only be cured with BMT.

May Hegglin anomaly and variants of *Alport's syndrome* are both characterised by giant platelets. The former is a benign condition, but the latter is associated with progressive hereditary nephritis and deafness.

Glanzmann's thrombasthenia, the Bernard-Soulier syndrome and platelet-type von Willebrand's disease are characterised by absence or abnormalities of platelet membrane glycoproteins resulting in defective platelet adhesion and aggregation.

In *platelet storage pool diseases* deficiencies in either the α or dense granules cause poor secondary platelet aggregation. There are also a variety of further specific surface membrane defects and internal enzyme abnormalities, which although difficult to define, can cause troublesome chronic bleeding problems.

Acquired abnormalities

Decreased production of platelets due to suppression or failure of the bone marrow is the commonest cause of thrombocytopenia. In aplastic anaemia, leukaemia and marrow infiltration, and after chemotherapy, thrombocytopenia is usually associated with a failure of red and white cell production but may be an isolated finding secondary to drug toxicity (penicillamine, cotrimoxazole), alcohol, or viral infection (HIV, infectious mononucleosis). Viral infection is the most common cause of mild transient thrombocytopenia.

Increased platelet consumption may be due to immune or non-immune mechanisms. *Idiopathic thrombocytopenic purpura (ITP)* is a relatively common disorder and is the most frequent cause of an isolated thrombocytopenia without anaemia or neutropenia. In adults it often presents insidiously, most frequently in women aged 15-50 years and can be associated with other autoimmune diseases, in particular systemic lupus erythematosus or the primary antiphospholipid syndrome. In children the onset is more acute and often follows a viral infection. The autoantibody produced is usually IgG, directed against antigens on the platelet membrane. Antibody-coated platelets are removed by the reticuloendothelial system, reducing the life span of the platelet to a few hours. The platelet count can vary from $<5 \times 10^9/l$ to near normal. The severity of bleeding is less than that seen with comparable degrees of thrombocytopenia in bone marrow failure due to the predominance of young, larger, and functionally superior platelets.

Post-transfusion purpura (PTP) is a rare complication of blood transfusion. It presents with severe thrombocytopenia 7-10 days after the transfusion and usually occurs in multiparous women who are negative for the human platelet antigen 1a (HPA1a). Antibodies to HPA1a develop, and in some way this alloantibody is responsible for the immune destruction of autologous platelets.

Neonatal alloimmune thrombocytopenia (NAITP) is similar to haemolytic disease of the newborn except that the antigenic stimulus comes from platelet specific antigens rather than red cell antigens. In 80% of cases the antigen is human platelet antigen 1a, and mothers negative (about 5% of the population) for this antigen form antibodies when sensitised by a fetus positive for the antigen. Fetal platelet destruction results from transplacental passage of these antibodies and severe bleeding, including intracranial haemorrhage, can occur in utero.

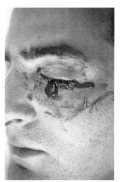

Figure 7.4 Bleeding around the eye in a patient with Bernard-Soulier syndrome

Box 7.1 Acquired disorders of reduced platelet production due to bone marrow failure or replacement
- Drug induced
- Leukaemia
- Metastatic tumour
- Aplastic anaemia
- Myelodysplasia
- Cytotoxic drugs
- Radiotherapy
- Associated with infection
- Megaloblastic anaemia

Diseases of the platelet storage pool are deficiencies in either the α or dense granules causing poor secondary platelet aggregation

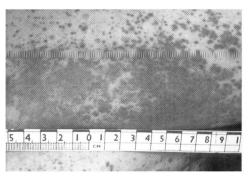

Figure 7.5 Spontaneous skin purpura in severe immune thrombocytopenia

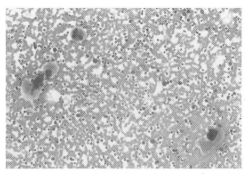

Figure 7.6 Bone marrow aspirate showing increased megakaryocytes in immune thrombocytopenia

Firstborns are frequently affected and successive pregnancies are equally or more affected.

Heparin-induced thrombocytopenia (HIT) occurs during unfractionated heparin therapy in up to 5% of patients, but is less frequently associated with low molecular weight heparins. It may become manifest when arterial or venous thrombosis occurs during a fall in the platelet count and is thought to be due to the formation of antibodies to heparin that are bound to platelet factor 4, a platelet granule protein. The immune complexes activate platelets and endothelial cells, resulting in thrombocytopenia and thrombosis coexisting. Heparin-induced thrombocytopenia carries an appreciable mortality risk if the diagnosis is delayed.

In thrombotic thrombocytopenic purpura (TTP) the presenting features can be fever, fluctuating neurological signs, renal impairment, and intravascular haemolysis, resulting in thrombocytopenia. Recent evidence suggests that the condition is caused by an autoantibody to a protease enzyme which is responsible for cleaving the ultra-high molecular weight multimers of von Willebrand factor. The development of this antibody causes a circulating excess of highly active multimers, causing intravascular platelet agglutination in vivo and the precipitation of a microangiopathic haemolytic anaemia. The condition is suspected clinically by thrombocytopenia, red cell fragmentation on the blood film, and a reticulocytosis. The demonstration of an abnormal pattern of von Willebrand multimers will make the diagnosis highly likely and the complete absence of the cleaving protease caused by an inhibitory antibody can be proved in some specialised laboratories.

Disseminated intravascular coagulation usually occurs in critically ill patients as a result of catastrophic activation of the coagulation pathway, often due to sepsis. Widespread platelet consumption occurs causing thrombocytopenia.

The spleen normally pools about a third of the platelet mass, but in massive splenomegaly this can increase up to 90%, resulting in apparent thrombocytopenia.

Aspirin, non-steroidal anti-inflammatory agents, and glycoprotein IIb/IIIa antagonists are the most common cause of acquired platelet dysfunction. For this reason aspirin and the IIb/IIIa antagonists are used therapeutically as antiplatelet agents. Aspirin acts by irreversibly inhibiting cyclo-oxygenase activity in the platelet, resulting in impairment of the granule release reaction and defective aggregation. The effects of a single dose of aspirin last for the lifetime of the platelet (7-10 days). Clopidogrel, a thienopyridine derivative, has now been introduced as an oral antiplatelet agent which inhibits ADP binding to the platelet membrane and is useful in patients who are intolerant or resistant to aspirin. It is becoming widely used as a prophylactic agent for myocardial ischaemia and related coronary syndromes.

Bleeding in uraemic patients is most commonly from defects in platelet adhesion or aggregation, though thrombocytopenia, severe anaemia with packed cell volume <20% or coagulation defects can also contribute.

In essential (primary) thrombocytosis (ET) and *reactive (secondary) thrombocytosis* the platelet count is raised above the upper limit of normal. A wide range of disorders can cause a raised platelet count ($>800 \times 10^9$/l), but patients are normally asymptomatic, except in ET, when excessive spontaneous bleeding may develop when the count exceeds 1000×10^9/l. Antiplatelet drugs can be useful to prevent thrombosis in high risk patients, for example, postoperatively. Some myelodysplastic syndromes may be complicated by an acquired storage pool type platelet disorder.

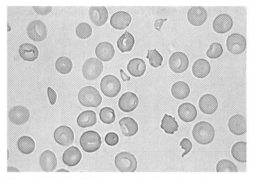

Figure 7.7 Red cell fragmentation in patient who presented with confusion and lethargy in whom thrombotic thrombocytopenic purpura was diagnosed. She responded well to large volume plasma exchange for one week

Box 7.2 Post-transfusion purpura

- This is an acquired abnormality
- It is a rare complication of blood transfusion presenting with severe thrombocytopenia 7-10 days after the transfusion
- Patients are usually multiparous women who are negative for the human platelet antigen 1a
- Antibodies to this antigen develop that are somehow responsible for the immune destruction of the patient's own platelets

Box 7.3 Causes of acquired platelet dysfunction

- Aspirin and non-steroidal anti-inflammatory agents
- Penicillins and cephalosporins
- Uraemia
- Alcohol
- Liver disease
- Myeloproliferative disorders
- Myeloma
- Cardiopulmonary bypass
- Fish oils

Box 7.4 Disorders with increased consumption of platelets

- Disorders with immune mechanism
  Autoimmune: idiopathic thrombocytopenic purpura
  Alloimmune: post-transfusion purpura, neonatal alloimmune thrombocytopenia
  Infection associated: infectious mononucleosis, HIV, malaria
  Drug induced: heparin, penicillin, quinine, sulphonamides, rifampicin
- Thrombotic thrombocytopenic purpura/haemolytic uraemic syndrome
- Hypersplenism and splenomegaly
- Disseminated intravascular coagulation
- Massive transfusion

Box 7.5 Thrombocytosis

- Essential (primary) thrombocytosis
- Reactive (secondary) thrombocytosis
  Infection
  Malignant disease
  Acute and chronic inflammatory diseases
  Pregnancy
  After splenectomy
  Iron deficiency
  Haemorrhage

History and examination of patients

Abnormal bleeding associated with thrombocytopenia or abnormal platelet function is characterised by spontaneous skin purpura and ecchymoses, mucous membrane bleeding and protracted bleeding after trauma. Prolonged nose bleeds can occur, particularly in children, and menorrhagia or postpartum haemorrhage is common in women. Rarely, subconjunctival, retinal, gastrointestinal, genitourinary or intracranial bleeds may occur. In thrombocytopenic patients severe spontaneous bleeding is unusual with a platelet count $\geq 20 \times 10^9/l$.

Investigations

The investigations in a suspected platelet disorder will depend on the presentation and history in each patient. If the bleeding is severe the patient may need urgent hospital referral for prompt evaluation, diagnosis, and treatment, which may entail blood product support. All patients should have a full blood count, blood film, coagulation, and biochemical screen, followed by further investigations depending on the results of these.

Thrombocytopenia can be artefactual and due to platelet clumping or a blood clot in the sample, which should be excluded in all cases. The skin bleeding time, which is invasive, variable and not reliable in screening mild platelet disorders, has been replaced by devices which perform an in vitro bleeding time on small volumes of citrated blood and simulate platelet function in a high shear rate situation. The sensitivity of these devices for all platelet disorders is still under investigation.

Management

All serious bleeding due to a platelet disorder needs haematological assessment and treatment. Mild or trivial bleeding due to a transient postviral thrombocytopenia or aspirin ingestion needs no active treatment and can be managed in the community.

Congenital disorders

A neonate or small infant with bleeding must be referred for evaluation as the inherited bleeding disorders (eg haemophilia or von Willebrand's disease) and platelet disorders can present at a very young age.

Bleeding episodes in all the congenital thrombocytopenias and platelet function disorders require filtered HLA-compatible platelet transfusions to secure haemostasis, though in minor episodes in the dysfunctional syndromes desmopressin (DDAVP) given intravenously or intranasally with anti-fibrinolytics (tranexamic acid) may be sufficient. There is increasing evidence that in selected patients with congenital disorders recombinant factor VIIa may be of use in the treatment or prevention of bleeding. This avoids exposure to blood products but is expensive. Bone marrow transplantation can potentially offer a cure in a number of these conditions.

Acquired disorders

In thrombocytopenia due to bone marrow failure or marrow infiltration—for example leukaemia or cancer—prophylactic platelet transfusions are given to keep the platelet count above $10 \times 10^9/l$ though the threshold is higher in infected or bleeding patients or to cover invasive procedures.
In childhood idiopathic thrombocytopenic purpura spontaneous recovery is common, and treatment is given only

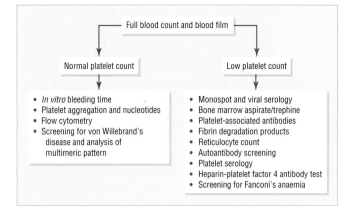

Figure 7.8 Investigation of suspected platelet disorder

A neonate or small infant with bleeding must be referred for evaluation as the inherited bleeding disorders (eg haemophilia or von Willebrand's disease) and platelet disorders may present at a very young age

Box 7.6 Treatment of platelet disorders

Congenital disorders
- Platelet transfusions (leucodepleted, HLA compatible and irradiated)
- DDAVP
- Tranexamic acid
- Recombinant factor VIIa
- Bone marrow transplantation

Acquired disorders
- Bone marrow failure
    Platelet transfusions if platelet count $<10 \times 10^9/l$
- Idiopathic thrombocytopenic purpura (adults)
    Prednisolone
    Intravenous immunoglobulin
    Splenectomy
- Post-transfusion purpura
    Intravenous immunoglobulin
    Plasma exchange
- Heparin-induced thrombocytopenia
    Anticoagulation but without heparin
- Thrombotic thrombocytopenic purpura
    Large volume plasma exchange
    Aspirin when platelets $>50 \times 10^9/l$
- Disseminated intravascular coagulation
    Treat underlying cause
    Fresh frozen plasma
    Platelet transfusion
- Hypersplenism
    Splenectomy if severe
- Platelet function disorders
    Platelet transfusion
    DDAVP (occasionally of use; for example in uraemia)

ABC of Clinical Haematology

in life-threatening bleeding. In adults the condition rarely
remits without treatment and is more likely to become chronic.
Initial treatment is prednisolone 1 mg/kg daily (80% of cases
remit) or intravenous immunoglobulin (0.4 g/kg for five days
or 1 g/kg for two days), or both combined. In refractory
patients splenectomy has a 60-70% chance of long term cure
and azathioprine, danazol, vinca alkaloids and high dose
dexamethasone have all been tried with variable success. Post-
transfusion purpura may respond to intravenous
immunoglobulin (at doses given above), or plasma exchange
may be required. Platelet transfusions should be avoided.
Patients in whom heparin-induced thrombocytopenia is
suspected are often inpatients with ongoing thrombosis and
may have complex medical problems. It is essential to withdraw
heparin and treat thrombosis with other anticoagulants,
avoiding all forms of heparin. Warfarin, synthetic heparinoids
or ancrod can be used. Platelet transfusions are contraindicated
in heparin-induced thrombocytopenia and in thrombotic
thrombocytopenic purpura. If the latter is suspected clinically
and on the basis of laboratory tests, large volume plasma
exchange should be started immediately and continued daily
until there is substantial clinical improvement, and all the
results of haematological tests have normalised. Aspirin can be
started once the platelet count is $>50 \times 10^9/l$.

With disseminated intravascular coagulation it is essential to
treat the underlying cause as well as support depletion of
clotting factors and platelets with blood products.

In pronounced bleeding or risk of bleeding due to the
acquired disorders of platelet function, platelets usually have to
be transfused to provide normally functioning platelets, though
desmopressin (DDAVP) and tranexamic acid can also be of
value. Usually treatment may only be necessary to cover surgical
procedures or major haemorrhage.

Further reading
- Coller BS. Anti-GPIIb/IIIa drugs: current strategies and future directions. *Thromb Haemostas* 2001;86:427-43.
- Hardistry RM. Platelet functional disorders. In: Lilleyman J, Hann I, Blanchette V, eds. *Pediatric hematology*, 2nd edn. Edinburgh: Churchill Livingstone, 2000.
- Rendu F, Brohard-Bohn B. The platelet release reaction: granules' constituents, secretion and functions. *Platelets* 2001;12:261-73.
- Shapiro AD. Platelet function disorders. *Haemophilia* 2000;6: 120-7.
- Smith OP. Inherited and congenital thrombocytopenia. In: Lilleyman J, Hann I, Blanchette V, eds. *Pediatric hematology*, 2nd edn. Edinburgh: Churchill Livingstone, 2000.

32

8 The myelodysplastic syndromes

David G Oscier

The term myelodysplastic syndromes was introduced in 1975 by a group of French, American, and British haematologists (FAB group) to describe a group of disorders with characteristic abnormalities of peripheral blood and bone marrow morphology and impaired bone marrow function, which tend to evolve into acute myeloid leukaemia. Although the myelodysplastic syndromes may occur at any age, they are predominantly diseases of elderly people.

Aetiology and pathogenesis

Primary myelodysplastic syndrome describes those cases—the majority—in which the cause is unknown. Case-control studies have shown a modest correlation between the myelodysplastic syndromes and exposure to low doses of radiation and organic chemicals.

Therapy-related myelodysplastic syndrome, sometimes called secondary myelodysplastic syndrome, describes cases that have arisen as a long term complication of cytotoxic chemotherapy, radiotherapy and particularly following autologous transplantation for lymphoma. The risk is highest 4-10 years after treatment with alkylating agents, such as chlorambucil and cyclophosphamide.

The hypothesis that patients who develop myelodysplastic syndrome following chemotherapy or exposure to environmental toxins may have inherited an impaired ability to metabolise and detoxify potential carcinogens or repair DNA damage is currently being investigated.

The combination of peripheral blood cytopenias and a hypercellular bone marrow found in the majority of patients with myelodysplastic syndromes can be explained by an increased susceptibility to apoptosis (programmed cell death) of bone marrow precursor cells. Immune mediated T cell myelosuppression results in marrow hypocellularity in the remaining 10-20% of patients.

Diagnosis

Patients present with the features of bone marrow failure—namely, symptoms of anaemia, bacterial infections, and bleeding or bruising. Splenomegaly is present in about 10% of patients, particularly in chronic myelomonocytic leukaemia, one subtype of the myelodysplastic syndromes. Increasingly, myelodysplastic syndrome is an incidental finding in elderly patients whose routine blood count shows an unexplained anaemia, macrocytosis, neutropenia, monocytosis, or thrombocytopenia.

The myelodysplastic syndromes can be diagnosed only by a haematologist, primarily on the basis of characteristic full blood count indices, morphological abnormalities on the peripheral blood film, and characteristic bone marrow appearances. Although myelodysplastic syndrome may sometimes be diagnosed on the basis of a blood film alone, a bone marrow aspirate and trephine are necessary to make a confident diagnosis and to assess the severity of the disease. Marrow examination can safely be omitted only in elderly, infirm patients with mild cytopenias who would not need treatment regardless of the marrow findings.

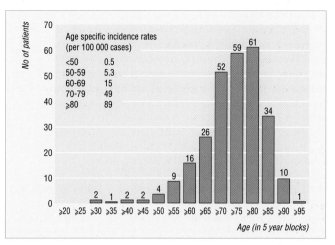

Figure 8.1 Age distribution and incidence rates per 1 000 000 population of patients presenting with myelodysplastic syndrome in Bournemouth, 1981-90

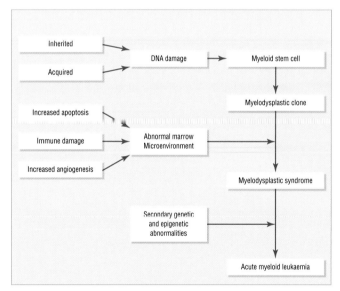

Figure 8.2 Pathogenesis of myelodysplastic syndrome

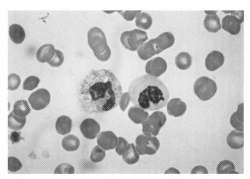

Figure 8.3 Blood film showing normal neutrophil (left) and dysplastic neutrophil with granular cytoplasm and hypolobated nucleus

Diagnosis is frequently straightforward, particularly if morphological abnormalities are found in the three major lineages—erythroid (red cells), myeloid (granulocytes, including neutrophils), and megakaryocytic series (platelets)—in the clinical context of an elderly patient with a peripheral blood cytopenia. However, morphological dysplasia is not synonymous with myelodysplastic syndrome, and similar morphological abnormalities to those found in early myelodysplastic syndromes may be seen in vitamin B_{12} deficiency or folate deficiency, alcohol excess, after cytotoxic chemotherapy, HIV infection, and even in a minority of cells in the bone marrow of normal individuals. Problems also arise if morphological abnormalities are subtle, if they involve only one cell lineage, or if the staining of blood and marrow slides is suboptimal.

Chromosome analysis

Cytogenetic analysis should be performed in all cases in which bone marrow examination is indicated. It is valuable both prognostically and when the morphological diagnosis is difficult. A clonal chromosome abnormality—that is, the same abnormality appearing in more than one cell—confirms the presence of a primary bone marrow disorder and excludes the reactive causes of dysplasia listed above. Chromosomal abnormalities are found in 30-50% of cases of primary myelodysplastic syndrome and in 80% of cases of therapy-related myelodysplastic syndrome. Specific chromosomal abnormalities may be associated with particular clinical and haematological features. For example, loss of part of a long arm ("q") of chromosome 5 occurring as the only chromosomal abnormality (5q- syndrome) is associated with macrocytic anaemia in elderly women and a low risk of transformation to acute myeloid leukaemia. Loss of the short arm ("p") of chromosome 17 is found in advanced disease and is associated with drug resistance and short survival.

The recent introduction of new and more powerful techniques to detect genetic abnormalities and study both gene and protein expression should lead to the identification of the key genetic events which initiate myelodysplastic syndromes and result in disease progression and evolution to acute leukaemia.

Table 8.2 Chromosome abnormalities in myelodysplasia

Abnormality	Incidence(%)	
	Primary myelodysplastic syndrome	Therapy related myelodysplastic syndrome
Deletion of 5q	10-20	20
Monosomy 7	10-15	30-50
Trisomy 8	15	10
Loss of 17p	3	10

Classification

In 1982 the FAB group divided the myelodysplastic syndromes into five subgroups based on (a) the percentage of immature myeloid cells (blast cells) and ring sideroblasts (immature red cells with iron granules arranged in a ring around the nucleus) in the bone marrow and (b) the presence or absence of a raised peripheral blood monocyte count. This classification was rapidly adopted worldwide and had prognostic significance. The World Health Organization (WHO) has now proposed

Table 8.1 Morphological abnormalities in myelodysplastic syndrome

Lineage	Blood	Marrow
Erythroid	Oval macrocytes	Abnormal nuclear shape and chromatin chromatin pattern
	Basophilic stippling	Ring sideroblasts
Myeloid	Hypogranular neutrophils	
	Hypolobated neutrophil nuclei	
Megakaryocytic	Agranular platelets	Micromegakaryocytes Mononuclear megakaryocytes Megakaryocytes with separated nuclei

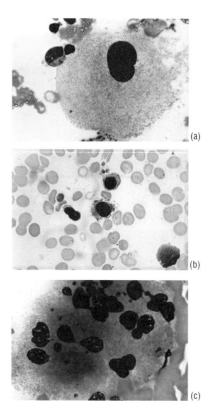

Figure 8.4 Abnormal megakaryocytes: (a) large mononuclear megakaryocyte; (b)micro megakaryocytes; (c) large polyploid megakaryocyte

Table 8.3 FAB classification of myelodysplastic syndrome

Category	Main criteria	Median survival (months)
Refractory anaemia (RA)	<5% marrow blasts	37
Refractory anaemia with ring sideroblasts (RARS)	<5% marrow blasts >15% ring sideroblasts	50
Refractory anaemia with excess blasts (RAEB)	5-20% marrow blasts	12
Refractory anaemia with excess blasts in transformation (RAEBt)	20-30% marrow blasts	5
Chronic myelomonocyte leukaemia (CMML)	$>1 \times 10^9$/l circulating monocytes <20% marrow blasts	19

Table 8.4 WHO classification of myelodysplastic syndrome

Category	Main criteria	Median survival (months)
Refractory anaemia (RA)	Erythroid dysplasia only <5% marrow blasts	69
Refractory anaemia with ring sideroblasts (RARS)	Erythroid dysplasia only <5% marrow blasts >15% ring sideroblasts	69
Refractory cytopenia with multilineage dysplasia (RCMD)	Bi- or tri-lineage dysplasia <5% marrow blasts	33
Refractory cytopenia with multilineage dysplasia and ring sideroblasts (RCMD)	Bi-or tri-lineage dysplasia <5% marrow blasts >15% ring sideroblasts	32
MDS associated with isolated del (5q) chromosome abnormality	Hypolobated megakaryocytes <5% marrow blasts Isolated del (5q)	116
Refractory anaemia with excess blasts (RAEB)	RAEB 1 5-9% marrow blasts RAEB 2 10-19% marrow blasts	18 10

a new classification based also on the percentage of blast cells and ring sideroblasts and also whether the dysplasia is uni- or multi-lineage, the presence of a particular cytogenetic abnormality and clinical course. Patients with more than 20% blasts in the bone marrow are considered to have acute leukaemia. Chronic myelomonocytic leukaemia is now classified as a mixed myelodysplastic/myeloproliferative disease, as many patients with CMML have features such as leucocytosis and splenomegaly which are more typical of a myeloproliferative disorder.

Natural course and prognosis

The clinical course of the myelodysplastic syndromes is extremely variable even among patients of the same subgroup. About two-thirds of patients die of marrow failure (of whom half undergo leukaemic transformation), and one-third die of unrelated causes. The median survival of patients with myelodysplastic syndrome is 20 months and for all subtypes is shorter than that of age matched controls.

Although both the FAB and WHO classifications have prognostic significance, a more accurate prediction of survival can be achieved by using an International Prognostic Scoring System (IPSS) which incorporates the presenting haemoglobin concentration, neutrophil and platelet counts, the percentage of blasts in the bone marrow, and chromosome abnormalities.

Management

The treatment of the myelodysplastic syndromes is generally unsatisfactory, which partially accounts for the variety of therapeutic options.

Before the most appropriate treatment can be determined, several factors must be taken into consideration. These include the patient's age and general fitness, the severity of the disease at presentation, prognostic factors, and whether the disease is stable or progressive. Consequently, whenever possible there should be a period of observation before a decision about long term treatment is made. In addition, management decisions should not be based on blood and bone marrow samples taken during severe bacterial infections as infections can result in acute and reversible changes in the neutrophil and platelet counts and the percentage of marrow blasts.

For most patients treatment is palliative, and the possibility of cure applies only to the minority of young patients suitable

Table 8.5 International prognostic scoring system

	Score value				
	0	0.5	1.0	1.5	2.0
BM blasts%	<5	5-10		11-20	21-30
Karyotype	Good	Int.	Poor		
Cytopenias	0/1	2/3			

Karyotype: Good, normal, -Y, del(5q), del(20q); Poor, complex (>3 abnormalities) or chromosome 7 anomalies; Int. = Intermediate, other abnormalities.

Cytopenias defined as haemoglobin concentration <10g/dl, neutrophils $<1.5 \times 10^9$/l and platelets $<100 \times 10^9$/l.

Table 8.6 Median survival of primary myelodysplastic syndrome using the IPSS score

Risk group	IPSS score	Median survial (yr)			
		<60	>60	<70	>70
Low	0	11.8	4.8	9	3.9
Int. 1	0.5-1.0	5.2	2.7	4.4	2.4
Int. 2	1.5-2.0	1.8	1.1	1.3	1.2
High	≥2.5	0.3	0.5	0.4	0.4

Int. = Intermediate

Box 8.1 Treatment options in myelodysplastic syndrome

- Observation
- Supportive care
  - Red cell and/or platelet transfusions
  - Antibiotics
  - Haemopoietic growth factors
- Immunosuppressive therapy
- Low dose chemotherapy
- Intensive chemotherapy
- Transplantation
  - Autologous
  - Allogeneic
    - Myeloablative
    - Non-myeloablative

for an allogeneic bone marrow transplant. Sixty per cent of such patients without an increase in marrow blasts and 40% of patients with increased blasts will be free of disease five years after transplantation. Non-myeloablative transplantation which utilises less intensive pretransplant chemotherapy and relies on a graft versus leukaemia effect to eradicate the malignant clone, significantly reduces transplant-related mortality. If ongoing studies demonstrate both longer term safety and efficacy then this procedure could be considered for patients up to the age of 65 years providing a suitable donor is available.

Patients with low risk disease defined by the International Prognostic Scoring System require observation only. The option of allogeneic transplantation should be discussed with intermediate I patients under the age of 65 years. Cytopenic patients who either decline or are unsuitable for transplantation may respond to immunosuppressive therapy with anti-lymphocyte globulin or cyclosporin, particularly if the bone marrow is hypocellular. Patients in the intermediate II and high risk groups under the age of 65 should be considered for intensive chemotherapy and responders then offered a transplant procedure since the median duration of response to chemotherapy alone is 12-18 months.

It should be stressed that all active treatment for the myelodysplastic syndrome and particularly transplant procedures should be conducted within clinical trials wherever possible.

Low dose cytotoxic treatment with hydroxyurea or etoposide may reduce spleen size and improve the blood count in patients with intermediate and poor risk chronic myelomonocytic leukaemia, but the median survival remains poor at less than two years.

The cornerstone of treatment remains the judicious use of red cells and platelet transfusions and antibiotics for most elderly patients with symptomatic disease. Iron chelation therapy should be considered for patients who need red cell transfusion long term. Recombinant growth factors have been used to treat both neutropenia and anaemia in the myelodysplastic syndromes. Granulocyte-colony stimulating factor (G-CSF) induces a transient neutrophilia in the majority of cases but long term intermittent G-CSF should only be considered for patients with severe neutropenia and recurrent infections. Erythropoietin can raise the haemoglobin and improve quality of life in some patients with myelodysplastic syndromes with <10% of bone marrow blasts. The addition of G-CSF improves the response rate, particularly in patients with ring sideroblasts. Response rates of 70% are achievable in patients with low basal erythropoietin levels and a transfusion requirement of <2 units per month. Growth factors are expensive, however, and the least effective in patients with advanced disease and severe cytopenias—those who most require treatment.

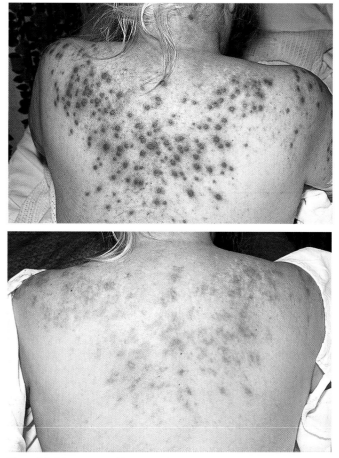

Figure 8.5 Seventy year old woman with refractory anaemia with excess blasts in transformation showing improvement in leukaemic skin deposits after course of low dose cytosine arabinoside

Further reading
- Bunning RD, Bennet JM, Flandrin G *et al.* Myelodysplastic syndromes. In: Jaffe ES *et al.*, eds. *WHO classification of tumours.* Lyon: IARC Press, 2001.
- Emanuel PD. Myelodysplasia and myelopreoliferative disorders in childhood: an update. *Br J Haematol* 1999;105:852-63.
- Germing U, Gattermann N, Strupp C *et al.* Validation of WHO proposals for a new classification of primary myelodysplastic syndromes: a retrospective analysis of 1600 patients. *Leukaemia Res* 2000;24:983-92.
- Hellstrom-Lindberg E, Negrin R, Stein R *et al.* Erythroid response to treatment with G-CSF plus erythropoietin for the anaemia of patients with myelodysplastic syndromes: proposal for a predictive model. *Br J Haematol* 1997;99:344-51.
- Molldrem J, Caples M, Mavroudis D *et al.* Antithymocyte globulin for patients with myelodysplastic syndrome. *Br J Haematol* 1997;99:699-705.
- Pedersen-Bjergaard J, Andersen M, Christiansen D. Therapy-related acute myeloid leukaemia and myelodysplasia after high dose chemotherapy and autologous stem cell transplantation. *Blood* 2000;95:3273-9.
- Witte T, Suciu S, Verhoef G *et al.* Intensive chemotherapy followed by allogeneic or autologous stem cell transplantation for patients with myelodysplastic syndromes (MDSs) and acute myeloid leukaemia following MDS. *Blood* 2001;98:2326-31.

The histogram showing age distribution and incidence rates for myelodysplastic syndrome is adapted with permission from the *British Journal of Haematology* (Williamson PJ, Kruger AR, Reynolds PJ, Hamblin TJ, Oscier DG. Establishing the incidence of myelodysplastic syndrome. 1994;87:743-5).

9 Multiple myeloma and related conditions

Charles R J Singer

A heterogeneous group of conditions are associated with monoclonal immunoglobulin (M protein or paraprotein) in the serum or urine and are characterised by disordered proliferation of monoclonal lymphocytes or plasma cells. The clinical phenotype of each condition is determined by the rate of accumulation, site and biological properties of the abnormal cells and also by the biological properties of the monoclonal protein.

Multiple myeloma

The incidence of myeloma is about 4 per 100 000 in Britain. It occurs more than twice as frequently in African Americans than in white Americans and Europeans, although it is much less common among Chinese and Japanese Asians. Myeloma is extremely rare in people aged under 40 years, but its incidence increases to over 30 per 100 000 in those aged over 80. The median age at diagnosis is 69 years, with slight male predominance.

Pathogenesis and clinical features

Myeloma is a tumour of monoclonal plasma cells that accumulate in the marrow, leading to anaemia, bone marrow failure and bone destruction. Immunoglobulin heavy chain analysis reveals that the tumour arises in a post-germinal centre B lymphocyte. This probably occurs in a lymph node or in the spleen and neoplastic cells home to the bone marrow, where the environment stimulates proliferation of plasma cells.

Most myeloma cells produce and secrete a monoclonal protein, usually intact immunoglobulin. IgG paraprotein is present in 60% of cases and IgA in 20-25%, and in 15-20% of cases free immunoglobulin light chains alone are produced. Myeloma in which the cells secrete IgD, two clonal proteins, IgM, or no protein at all are rare. Free light chains are detectable in urine as Bence Jones protein.

Accumulation of M protein may lead to hyperviscosity (especially IgA and IgM due to the size of the Ig molecule) or deposition of the protein in renal tubules, resulting in renal failure. Production of normal immunoglobulin is often depressed (immune paresis) and contributes to the patient's susceptibility to infection.

Bone destruction is a characteristic feature of myeloma, and the associated bone pain is a major cause of morbidity in myeloma. Myeloma is associated with abnormal bone remodelling due to increased osteoclastic bone resorption and inhibition of osteoblastic bone formation. This results in pronounced bone loss and the characteristic osteolytic lesions predisposing to pathological fractures. Widespread bone destruction may lead to hypercalcaemia, resulting in a vicious cycle of dehydration, worsening hypercalcaemia, and renal failure.

Interactions between marrow stroma cells (including osteoclasts) and myeloma cells play a critical role in myeloma cell proliferation and the development of bone disease. Stroma cells produce interleukin-6, a growth factor for myeloma cells, which in turn produce tumour necrosis factor α and interleukin-1 β. These stimulate stroma cell production of RANK-L (receptor activator of NFκ-B ligand). Binding of RANK-L to its receptor (RANK) expressed by osteoclast

Box 9.1 Conditions associated with M proteins

Stable production
- Monoclonal gammopathy of undetermined significance
- Smouldering multiple myeloma

Progressive production
- Multiple myeloma (IgG, IgA, free light chains, IgD, IgE, non-secretory, IgM)
- Plasma cell leukaemia
- Solitary plasmacytoma of bone
- Extramedullary plasmacytoma
- Waldenström's macroglobulinaemia (IgM)
- Chronic lymphocytic leukaemia
- Malignant lymphoma
- Primary amyloidosis
- Heavy chain disease

Box 9.2 Clinical features of myeloma

Common
- Bone pain and pathological fractures
- Anaemia and bone marrow failure
- Infection due to immune paresis and neutropenia
- Renal impairment

Less common
- Acute hypercalcaemia
- Symptomatic hyperviscosity
- Neuropathy
- Amyloidosis
- Coagulopathy

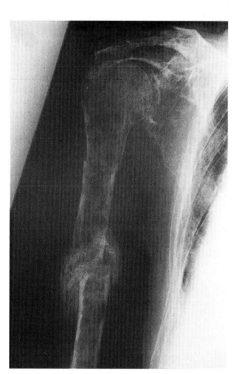

Figure 9.1 Radiograph showing multiple lytic lesions and pathological fractures of humerus

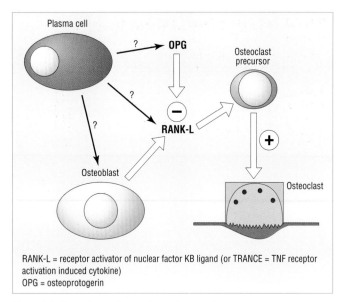

RANK-L = receptor activator of nuclear factor KB ligand (or TRANCE = TNF receptor activation induced cytokine)
OPG = osteoprotogerin

Figure 9.2 Osteoclast activation by myeloma cells

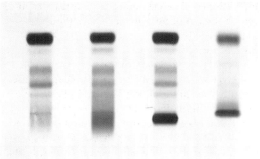

Figure 9.3 Protein electrophoresis strip showing (1) normal plasma, (2) polyclonal hypergammaglobulinaemia, (3) serum M protein, and (4) urine M protein (Bence Jones proteinuria) and albuminuria

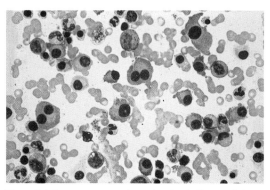

Figure 9.4 Bone marrow aspirate showing infiltrate of abnormal plasma cells (medium power)

precursors, promotes osteoclast proliferation and differentiation. Osteoprotogerin (OPG) is also produced by stroma cells, notably osteoblasts, which in experimental systems inhibits RANK-L binding and osteoclast formation. Osteoblasts are inhibited and secretion of OPG is reduced in myeloma.

Complex cytogenetic abnormalities are frequently found in myeloma using modern techniques. These most commonly involve chromosome 14q which is the site of the immunoglobulin heavy chain gene and deletions of chromosome 13 which confers an unfavourable prognosis.

The most common presenting complaint is bone pain (60%), commonly affecting the back. Symptoms of anaemia, renal failure, or infection are also frequent. Less common are symptoms of hyperviscosity (somnolence, impaired vision, purpura, and haemorrhage), acute hypercalcaemia, spinal cord compression, neuropathy, or amyloidosis. About 20% of patients are asymptomatic and detected through an elevated ESR or elevated globulin.

Investigations and diagnosis

Myeloma should be suspected in anyone aged over 40 years with unexplained bone pain or fractures, osteoporosis, osteolytic lesions, lethargy, anaemia, red cell rouleaux, raised erythrocyte sedimentation rate or plasma viscosity, hypercalcaemia, renal dysfunction, proteinuria, or recurrent infection. It is characterised by the triad of bone marrow plasmacytosis, lytic bone lesions on skeletal radiology, and the presence of M protein in the serum or urine or both. Not all patients have all these features and minimal diagnostic criteria have been established to assist with difficult cases.

History and examination should be followed by a full blood count and film; erythrocyte sedimentation rate or plasma viscosity; urea and creatinine concentrations; calcium, phosphate, and alkaline phosphatase concentrations; uric acid

Box 9.3 Minimal diagnostic criteria for myeloma

- >10% plasma cells in bone marrow or plasmacytoma on biopsy
- Clinical features of myeloma
- Plus at least one of:
  Serum paraprotein (IgG >30 g/l; IgA >20 g/l)
  Urine paraprotein (Bence Jones proteinuria)
  Osteolytic lesions on skeletal survey

Box 9.4 Investigation of patients with suspected myeloma

Useful screening tests
- Full blood count and film: anaemia often present; film may show rouleaux
- ESR or plasma viscosity: raised in the presence of a serum paraprotein
- Urea and creatinine: may indicate renal impairment
- Calcium, phosphate, alkaline phosphatase, and albumin: may reveal hypercalcaemia or low albumin
- Serum immunoglobulins: to detect immuneparesis
- Serum protein electrophoresis: to detect paraprotein
- Routine urinalysis: to detect proteinuria
- Urine electrophoresis for BJP: to detect paraprotein
- X-ray of sites of bone pain: may reveal pathological fracture or lytic lesion(s)

Diagnostic tests
- Bone marrow aspirate: to identify plasma cell infiltration
- Skeletal survey: to identify lytic bone lesions not already detected
- Paraprotein typing and quantification: to characterise paraprotein

Tests to establish tumour burden and prognosis
- Serum beta-2-microglobulin: measure of tumour load
- Serum C reactive protein: surrogate measure of IL-6
- Serum LDH: measure of tumour burden
- Serum albumin: when low reflects poor prognosis
- Cytogenetics: prognostic value

Tests that may be useful in some patients
- Creatinine clearance and 24 hour proteinuria
- MRI : not routine but useful in patients with cord compression or solitary plasmacytoma and abnormal in 30% of patients with normal skeletal survey
- CT : where clinically indicated
- Biopsy for amyloid and SAP scan: where suspected

concentration; serum protein electrophoresis; measurement of serum immunoglobulins; routine urine analysis; urine electrophoresis for Bence Jones protein; skeletal survey; and bone marrow aspirate and biopsy.

Normochromic normocytic anaemia is often present; neutropenia and thrombocytopenia suggest advanced disease. Rouleaux are usually seen in the blood film, and plasma cells may also be present in about 5% of cases. The erythrocyte sedimentation rate and plasma viscosity are often increased but are normal in 10% of cases. The serum calcium concentration is increased in up to 20% of cases. Serum alkaline phosphatase concentration is invariably normal, reflecting suppressed osteoblast activity. Raised urea and creatinine concentrations occur in 20% of case and renal impairment, usually due to cast nephropathy, is common. Low serum albumin concentration reflects advanced disease. Serum beta-2-microglobulin and C-reactive protein may be used to provide a prognostic index.

Skeletal radiology is a critical investigation and shows lytic lesions, pathological fracture or generalised bone rarefaction in 80% of cases. Only osteoporosis is seen in 5-10%. Bone scans are typically negative in multiple myeloma despite extensive bone damage and are of no value. Magnetic resonance imaging (MRI) is the most sensitive imaging technique for myeloma and is valuable in suspected cord compression. Although not routine it is useful in selected patients.

Approximately 10% of patients develop primary amyloid which causes nephrotic syndrome, renal and cardiac failure, and neuropathies. The extent of amyloid deposition can be assessed using serum amyloid P component (SAP) scanning procedures.

The most important differential diagnosis is between multiple myeloma and monoclonal gammopathy of undetermined significance for which no treatment is indicated. No single test differentiates the two conditions reliably. A serum IgG concentration >30g/l or IgA concentration >20g/l suggests a diagnosis of myeloma rather than monoclonal gammopathy of undetermined significance. The term "smouldering multiple myeloma" has been used for patients in whom M protein and bone marrow criteria exist for the diagnosis of myeloma, but anaemia, renal impairment, and skeletal lesions do not develop and crucially, the M protein and plasma cells remain stable. Here too a "watch and wait" policy is appropriate.

Several prognostic features have been recognised. Deletion of chromosome 13q is an important adverse feature. Renal impairment is a risk factor due to its association with a high tumour burden.

Management and clinical course

Without treatment, a patient with multiple myeloma is likely to experience progressive bone damage, anaemia and renal failure. Initial management should prioritise general aspects of care.

Infection is the most common cause of death. Initial treatment should consist of (a) adequate analgesia—opiates often, and local radiotherapy to fractures or osteolytic lesions may have dramatic benefit; (b) rehydration—patients are often dehydrated at presentation, even without hypercalcaemia or renal impairment; (c) management of hypercalcaemia if present—rehydration, diuresis, and bisphosphonate therapy; (d) management of renal impairment—rehydration and treatment of any hypercalcaemia often have a pronounced effect on abnormal serum chemistry in myeloma, though in some patients plasmapheresis and chemotherapy alone or with dialysis is effective; (e) treatment of infection—most infections at diagnosis are bacterial and respiratory and respond to broad

---

Box 9.5 Laboratory findings at diagnosis (proportion of cases)

• Normochromic normocytic anaemia	60%
• Increased erythrocyte sedimentation rate or plasma viscosity	90%
• Serum M protein	80%
• Urine M protein only	20%
• Raised serum calcium concentration	20%
• Raised serum creatinine concentration	25%
• Proteinuria	70%

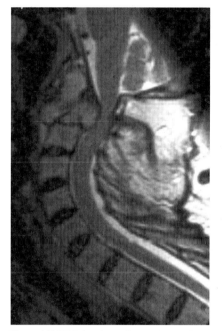

Figure 9.5 MRI showing collapse of second cervical vertebra and narrowing of spinal canal

---

Box 9.6 Features of poor prognosis at diagnosis

- Low haemoglobin concentration (<85 g/l)
- Hypercalcaemia
- Advanced lytic bone lesions
- High M protein production rates (IgG >70 g/l; IgA >50 g/l; Bence Jones protein >12 g/24 h)
- Abnormal renal function
- High plasma cell proliferative index
- Low serum albumin concentration (<30 g/l)
- High beta-2-microglobulin concentration (>6 mg/ml)
- High CRP
- 13q deletion

spectrum antibiotics, though later in the disease antifungal treatment may be necessary; and (f) chemotherapy.

Oral melphalan and prednisolone administered for 4 days at intervals of 4-6 weeks produces >50% reduction in the M protein concentration in 50% of patients. The treatment is well tolerated, but complete responses are rare and maximal response generally requires 12 months of treatment. Most patients achieve a "plateau phase" where the M protein remains stable despite further therapy and continues to do so for a median period of 12-18 months after chemotherapy stops. The median survival is about three years. During plateau phase clinical and laboratory results should be reviewed at regular intervals to identify progression at the earliest opportunity. Further treatment with melphalan may induce another plateau phase if a durable first plateau has been achieved. This treatment approach is widely used for patients over 65. Weekly cyclophosphamide is tolerated by almost all patients, including the few who fail to tolerate melphalan.

Combination intravenous chemotherapeutic regimens may produce higher response rates (up to 70%) and may improve survival. Combination regimens may be more effective in younger patients with high tumour loads, though they may be more toxic in elderly patients. The VAD combination (vincristine, doxorubicin and dexamethasone) produces a high response rate (80%), is well tolerated in renal impairment, requires 4-6 months of treatment to achieve maximum response and produces a higher proportion of complete responses (up to 20%). This treatment is less toxic to haemopoietic progenitors than standard melphalan treatment or other alkylator-containing regimens and is therefore more widely used in patients under 65 in whom autologous stem cell collection is planned.

High dose melphalan and autologous stem cell transplantation after initial treatment with VAD produces a complete response in up to 75% of patients and prolongs survival but is not curative. It is generally applicable only to patients under 65. Complete remission is generally associated with prolonged survival. Median duration of CR is two years and median overall survival is five years with this approach.

Allogeneic bone marrow transplantation may cure myeloma but carries significant treatment-related morbidity and mortality. It is generally restricted to patients under 50 with a compatible sibling. This treatment offers a 33% chance of durable remission and possible cure, 33% chance of survival with recurrence and 33% risk of transplant-related mortality.

Plateau phase

Most patients achieve a stable partial response with standard melphalan therapy with >50% reduction in the M protein. In plateau phase cessation of chemotherapy is not followed by a rise in the M band or further signs of progression for many months (median 6-12). Maintenance interferon alfa may prolong the plateau phase by six months, but little evidence exists of improved survival. Bisphosphonate treatment reduces the rate of further bone damage and may have an additive analgesic effect in patients with pre-existing damage. A survival benefit has been demonstrated in clinical trials and may reflect an effect of this treatment on the bone marrow microenvironment.

Disease progression

With regular follow up, serological detection of disease allows chemotherapy to be restarted before new bone damage develops. In many patients several separate periods of plateau phase may be re-induced by chemotherapy. Inevitably, myeloma becomes resistant to melphalan; oral dexamethasone may

---

Box 9.7 General aspects of care

- Pain control
    Analgesia (caution with NSAIDs)
    Local radiotherapy
- Limitation of renal damage
    Good fluid intake
    Caution with nephrotoxic drugs including NSAIDs
    Rapid treatment of hypercalcaemia
- Hypercalcaemia
    Rehydration
    Intravenous bisphosphonate
- Bone disease
    Local radiotherapy
    Long term bisphosphonates
    Fixation of potential fractures
- Cord compression
    MRI scanning to localise lesions
    Local radiotherapy
- Anaemia
    Blood transfusion
    Erythropoietin
- Infection
    Vigorous antibiotic therapy
    Annual influenza vaccination
- Hyperviscosity syndrome
    Plasmapheresis
    Prompt chemotherapy

Box 9.8 Options for initial chemotherapy in myeloma

- Melphalan with or without prednisolone
- Infusional chemotherapy—vincristine and adriamycin infusion plus either dexamethasone or methylprednisolone
- Combination therapy—for example, adriamycin, carmustine, cyclophosphamide, and melphalan
- Weekly cyclophosphamide ("C weekly")

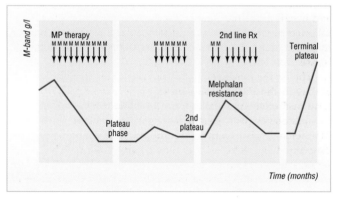

Figure 9.6 Natural history of multiple myeloma after melphalan treatment

achieve further responses, and oral low dose cyclophosphamide daily is often effective palliative treatment in combination with local radiotherapy to sites of bone pain. Thalidomide controls myeloma in over 20% of patients with advanced myeloma, and in combination with dexamethasone it achieves responses in up to 70% of patients previously treated with chemotherapy. Novel molecular therapies and derivatives of thalidomide show great potential.

Conditions related to multiple myeloma

Monoclonal gammopathy of undetermined significance

Monoclonal gammopathy of undetermined significance is defined by the presence of an M protein in a patient without multiple myeloma, Waldenström's macroglobulinaemia, amyloidosis, lymphoma, or other related disease. The prevalence of monoclonal gammopathy of undetermined significance is about 20 times greater than that of multiple myeloma, and the incidence increases with age (1% at over 50 years; 3% at over 70).

Multiple myeloma, macroglobulinaemia, amyloidosis, or lymphoma ultimately develops in 26% of patients with monoclonal gammopathy of undetermined significance, with an actuarial rate of 16% at 10 years.

Solitary plasmacytoma

About 5% of patients have a single bone lesion at diagnosis with no evidence of disseminated bone marrow involvement. Generally M protein is absent (up to 70% of cases) or present in low concentration. Plasmacytoma may be cured by local radiotherapy. Patients with solitary plasmacytoma should be monitored for evidence of myeloma, which develops in most cases. Further plasmacytomas may develop, and magnetic resonance imaging may show bone lesions undetectable by conventional radiology. Median survival is over 10 years.

Waldenström's macroglobulinaemia

This tumour is due to proliferation of lymphoid cells which produce monoclonal IgM. The median age at presentation is 63 years, and over 60% of patients are male. Many of the clinical features are due to hyperviscosity. Weakness, fatigue, and bleeding are the most common presenting complaints, followed by visual upset, weight loss, recurrent infections, dyspnoea, heart failure, and neurological symptoms. Bone pain is rare.

The erythrocyte sedimentation rate is greatly raised, and when the plasma viscosity exceeds 4 cP most patients have symptoms of hyperviscosity. Serum protein immunoelectrophoresis shows an IgM paraprotein. Monoclonal light chains may be present in the urine. Trephine biopsy often shows extensive infiltration with plasmacytoid lymphocytes.

Symptomatic hyperviscosity is corrected by plasmapheresis. Chlorambucil with or without prednisolone for one week every 4-6 weeks frequently reduces bone marrow infiltration, the IgM concentration, and plasma viscosity. Median survival is about five years. The purine analogue fludarabine is effective in this condition.

Other related conditions

Chronic lymphocytic leukaemia and diffuse low grade non-Hodgkin's lymphoma may be associated with low serum concentrations of monoclonal IgG or IgM. This finding has no prognostic importance for these patients. Primary amyloidosis

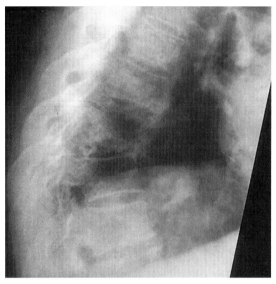

Figure 9.7 Bone pain from mechanical effects of myeloma damage (as in spine shown here) often necessitates long term treatment with strong analgesia despite response to chemotherapy

---

No treatment is indicated for monoclonal gammopathy of undetermined significance, but follow up is necessary

---

Box 9.9 Diagnostic criteria for monoclonal gammopathy of undetermined significance

- No unexplained symptoms suggestive of myeloma
- Serum M protein concentration <30 g/l
- <5% plasma cells in bone marrow
- Little or no M protein in urine
- No bone lesions
- No anaemia, hypercalcaemia, or renal impairment
- M protein concentration and other results stable on prolonged observation

---

Box 9.10 Plasma cell leukaemia

- May be diagnosed when blood plasma cells exceed $2.0 \times 10^9/l$
- May occur as a terminal stage in advanced multiple myeloma or as aggressive disease at diagnosis in under 5% of cases
- Bone involvement is often minimal, and the M protein concentration is often low
- Results of treatment are poor, intensive treatment can induce responses and prolong survival

---

Box 9.11 Clinical and laboratory features of Waldenström's macroglobulinaemia

- Fatigue and weight loss
- Anaemia
- Hyperviscosity syndrome (may cause chronic oral or nasal bleeding, visual upset, headache, vertigo, hearing loss, ataxia, somnolence, and coma)
- Retinal haemorrhages
- Venous congestion (sausage formation) in retinal veins
- Recurrent infection
- Lymphadenopathy
- Hepatosplenomegaly
- Raised erythrocyte sedimentation rate
- High serum monoclonal IgM concentration
- Lymphoplasmacytoid bone marrow infiltrate

Box 9.12 Key points
- In some cases distinguishing multiple myeloma from monoclonal gammopathy of undetermined significance can be difficult
- Prognostic factors are available which may help identify patients with myeloma in whom treatment may not be necessary, and others where aggressive treatment is warranted
- Early chemotherapy may reverse renal impairment and dialysis may be appropriate supportive therapy for some patients
- Bisphosphonate therapy helps reduce the incidence of bony complications
- Allogeneic bone marrow transplantation should be considered in younger myeloma patients (<55 years) if a compatible sibling donor is available since this may be curative

is associated with an M protein in 85%. The "heavy chain diseases" are rare lymphoproliferative disorders in which the abnormal cells excrete only parts of immunoglobulin heavy chains (γ, α, or μ).

Further reading
- Bataille R, Harrousseau JL. Multiple myeloma. *N Engl J Med* 1997;336:1657-64.
- Boccadoro M, Pileri A. Diagnosis, prognosis and standard treatment of multiple myeloma. *Hematol Oncol Clin North Am* 1997;11:111-31.
- Croucher PI, Apperley JF. Bone disease in multiple myeloma. *Br J Haematol* 1998;103:902-10.
- Fassas A, Tricot G. Results of high dose treatment with autologous stem cell support in patients with multiple myeloma. *Semin Hematol* 2001;38:231-42.
- Gahrton G, Svensson H, Cavo M *et al.* Progress in allogeneic bone marrow and peripheral blood stem cell transplantation for multiple myeloma: a comparison between transplants performed 1983-93 and 1994-8 at the European Group for Blood and Marrow Transplantation centres. *Br J Haematol* 2001;113:209-16.
- Gillmore JD, Hawkins PN, Pepys MB. Amyloidosis: a review of recent diagnostic and therapeutic developments. *Br J Haematol* 1997;99:245-56.
- Kyle RA. Monoclonal gammopathy of undetermined significance and solitary plasmacytoma. *Hematol Oncol Clin North Am* 1997;11:71-83.

Mr Darren Costello supplied the protein electrophoresis strip.

10 Bleeding disorders, thrombosis, and anticoagulation

K K Hampton, F E Preston

Blood within the vascular tree remains fluid throughout life, but if a blood vessel is damaged, blood will clot in a rapid localised response. Failure of clotting leads to bleeding disorders; thrombosis is inappropriate clotting within blood vessels. The haemostatic system is complex, and many congenital and acquired conditions can disturb its correct functioning.

Bleeding disorders

History
Personal and family history is as important as laboratory investigation in assessing bleeding disorders. Easy bruising, nosebleeds (especially in children), and menorrhagia are common and do not necessarily signify a haemostatic defect unless they are persistent and severe. Small bruises on the limbs in response to minor trauma and simple easy bruising are especially common in elderly people and those receiving long term corticosteroids.

Large bruises after minimal trauma and on the trunk may indicate an important haemostatic defect. Abnormally prolonged bleeding from minor cuts and scratches and delayed recurrence of bleeding are also important, as is gum bleeding if there is no gingival disease and if it is unrelated to the trauma of brushing. Repeated nosebleeds lasting more than 10 minutes despite compression suggest a local cause or an underlying bleeding disorder.

The haemostatic response to previous haemostatic challenges is informative, especially in mild conditions, when spontaneous bleeding is rare. A history of excessive bleeding or recurrence of bleeding after dental extractions, circumcision, tonsillectomy, other previous surgical operations, and childbirth should be sought, as should a history of unexplained anaemia, gastrointestinal bleeding without the demonstration of a cause, and previous blood transfusion.

A drug history should be taken to assess intake of aspirins and non-steroidal anti-inflammatory drugs, and appropriate questioning will suggest causes for acquired haemostatic disorders, such as excessive alcohol intake, liver disease, or renal disease.

An inherited bleeding condition will result in a family history of the condition and suggest a pattern of inheritance—for example, autosomal dominant inheritance (both sexes affected) or X-linked inheritance (only males affected).

In severe coagulation factor deficiency, such as haemophilia A or B, bleeding occurs primarily into muscles and joints, whereas in platelet disorders and von Willebrand's disease bleeding tends to be mucocutaneous—for example, nosebleeds, menorrhagia, and gum and gastrointestinal bleeding.

Laboratory investigation
The vast majority of important bleeding disorders can be excluded if the findings are all normal for blood and platelet counts, blood film, prothrombin time, activated partial thromboplastin time, fibrinogen or thrombin time, and bleeding time. These tests will reveal quantitative platelet disorders and congenital or acquired deficiency of coagulation

---

Box 10.1 History in bleeding disorders

- Abnormal bruising
- Abnormal bleeding from cuts and abrasions
- Nosebleeds
- Menorrhagia
- Haemarthrosis
- Bleeding after dental extraction
- Bleeding during childbirth
- Bleeding during surgery
- Previous anaemia and transfusions
- Drug history
- Family history

Persistent menorrhagia sufficient to cause iron deficiency anaemia may indicate a bleeding disorder if no structural uterine abnormality is present

---

Table 10.1 Screening tests for bleeding disorders

Test	Abnormality detected
Blood count and film	Anaemia, leukaemia, disseminated intravascular coagulation
Platelet count	Thrombocytopenia
Activated partial thromboplastin time	Deficiency of all coagulation factors except VII, especially follows VIII and IX; heparin
Prothrombin time	Deficiency of factors I, II, V, VII, and X; warfarin
Thrombin time or fibrinogen	Hypofibrinogenaemia or dysfibrinogenaemia; heparin; fibrin degradation products
Bleeding time	Test of platelet-vessel wall interaction

Patients who have unexplained abnormalities on screening investigations should be referred for specialist investigation and management

ABC of Clinical Haematology

factors, which can be confirmed by specific assay. The tests will not, however, detect all bleeding disorders, especially those due to vascular causes and mild von Willebrand's disease, and patients with a strong personal or family history of the condition, despite normal screening investigation, should be referred for specialist investigation and management.

Congenital disorders

Haemophilia A and B are rare conditions with a combined incidence of about 1:10 000 of the population. They are due to a deficiency of coagulation factors VIII (haemophilia A) and IX (haemophilia B). As the genes for both proteins are on the X chromosome, both haemophilias have sex-linked inheritance—the daughters of a man with haemophilia are therefore obligate carriers. Patients with severe haemophilia (less than 2% factor VIII or IX) have spontaneous bleeding into muscles and joints that can lead to a crippling arthropathy. Patients with moderate (2-5%) and mild (>5%) conditions usually bleed only after trauma or surgery. Management is highly specialised and consists of preventing or treating bleeding episodes with plasma-derived or recombinant clotting factors.

Von Willebrand's disease is a common bleeding disorder, with an incidence of up to 1% in some populations. Most cases are mild, with bleeding only after a haemostatic challenge. Menorrhagia is common in affected women. Inheritance is autosomal dominant, with males and females equally affected. The condition is due to a reduction or structural abnormality of von Willebrand factor, which has the dual role of promoting normal platelet function and stabilising coagulation factor VIII. Von Willebrand's disease can give normal results on screening tests, and diagnosis may require specialist investigation. Most patients with mild disease respond to desmopressin (DDAVP), but clotting factor concentrates are needed for a minority.

Acquired disorders

Most proteins of the coagulation cascade and their regulators and inhibitors necessary for haemostasis are synthesised in the liver. Acquired abnormalities can be due to impaired synthesis, increased consumption, or rarely the formation of autoantibodies against coagulation proteins. Liver disease can cause a severe bleeding disorder, with prolongation of the prothrombin time particularly, often with coexistent thrombocytopenia due to excessive pooling of platelets in an

Table 10.3 Clinical severity of haemophilia A and B

Factor value*	Bleeding tendency
<0.02	Severe—frequent spontaneous bleeding into joints, muscles, and internal organs
0.02-0.05	Moderate—some "spontaneous" bleeds, bleeding after minor trauma
>0.05	Mild—bleeding only after significant trauma or surgery

*Normal value of factors VIII and IX is 0.5-1.5

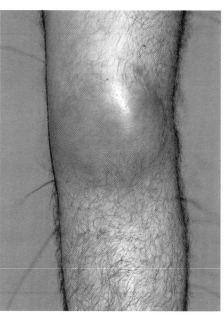

Figure 10.1 Acute haemarthrosis of knee joint

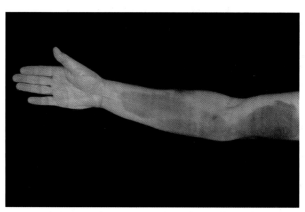

Figure 10.2 Pathological bruising in von Willebrand's disease

Table 10.2 Clinical features of coagulation factor deficiency and platelet type/von Willebrand's disease

	Coagulation defect	Platelet/von Willebrand's disease
Bruises	Large, on body and limbs	Small
Bleeding from cuts	Not severe	Profuse
Nosebleeds	Not common	Common, often prolonged and severe
Gastrointestinal bleeding	Uncommon, no underlying lesion	Common
Haemarthrosis	Common in severe haemophilia	Very uncommon
Haematuria	Common	Rare
Bleeding after dental extraction and surgery	Delayed 12-24 hours after haemostatic challenge	From time of challenge

Table 10.4 Acquired bleeding disorders

Disease	Pathophysiology
Liver disease and cirrhosis	Decreased synthesis of coagulation factors, thrombocytopenia
Gastrointestinal malabsorption	Vitamin K deficiency
Shock/sepsis/malignancy	Disseminated intravascular coagulation, increased consumption of coagulation factors and platelets
Renal disease	Acquired platelet dysfunction
Lymphoproliferative disorders/spontaneous	Acquired autoantibodies to specific coagulation factors (inhibitors)
Amyloidosis	Acquired factor X deficiency, blood vessel infiltration

enlarged spleen. Malabsorption of vitamin K from the gut can cause a coagulation disorder similar to that caused by ingestion of warfarin. Disseminated intravascular coagulation is a rare cause of an acquired severe systemic failure of haemostasis with simultaneous microvascular thrombosis and generalised bleeding. Overwhelming bacterial infections—for example, meningococcal septicaemia or disseminated malignancies (such as prostatic, pancreatic, and acute promyelocytic leukaemia)—are the most common causes. Renal disease causes a variable bleeding disorder primarily due to platelet dysfunction; advancing age, prolonged use of steroids, and vitamin C deficiency can all result in excessive bruising. Abnormal bleeding has been reported with myeloproliferative, myelodysplastic, and lymphoproliferative disorders.

Arterial thrombosis
Arterial thrombosis results in myocardial infarction, stroke, and peripheral vascular disease. Atherosclerotic lesions form in the vessel wall, resulting in narrowing and subsequent plaque rupture, which cause vessel occlusion. Risk factors for atherosclerosis include smoking, hypertension, diabetes, hypercholesterolaemia, hyperlipidaemia, and hyperfibrinogenaemia. Platelet deposition occurs on a ruptured arteriosclerotic plaque, and the antiplatelet drugs aspirin and clopidogrel are widely used in the treatment and secondary prophylaxis of arterial thrombosis.

Venous thrombosis
Venous thrombosis results in deep vein thrombosis and pulmonary embolism and is due to a combination of blood stasis and hypercoagulability. The clinical diagnosis of venous thromboembolic disease is notoriously unreliable, and objective confirmation with ultrasonography or venography for deep vein thrombosis and ventilation perfusion scanning or pulmonary angiography for pulmonary embolus must be performed. Recently it has become clear that venous thrombosis is frequently due to a combination of environmental factors (such as surgery and pregnancy), with an underlying genetic predisposition due to inherited deficiencies or abnormalities of the proteins of the natural anticoagulant pathway, which functions to inhibit or limit thrombin formation. The familial thrombophilic disorders include factor V Leiden, prothrombin 20210A and deficiencies of protein C, protein S, and antithrombin.

The incidence of factor V Leiden, which causes activated protein C resistance (APCR), is 3-5%, and that of the prothrombin 20210A allele is 2-3% in Caucasian populations. These are thus the commonest causes of an inherited predisposition to venous thrombosis (thrombophilia), despite being rare in other ethnic groups. All the hereditary thrombophilic conditions are autosomally dominantly inherited and are present in up to 50% of cases of venous thrombosis, particularly when recurrent, familial, or at a young age. Detection of one of these conditions may influence the future management of the individual with regard to thromboprophylaxis and anticoagulation.

Consideration should also be given to possible family screening. Unfortunately, the presence of active thrombosis and treatment with both heparin and warfarin make testing for the above deficiency conditions unreliable, and testing should be delayed until active thrombosis has resolved and anticoagulants have been discontinued. The genetic tests for the factor V Leiden defect and the prothrombin 20210A allele are, of course, unaffected by anticoagulant therapy and on-going thrombosis.

An acquired predisposition to both arterial and venous thrombosis occurs in the antiphospholipid syndrome, which

Box 10.2 Risk factors for venous thrombosis
Environmental
- Immobility
- Surgery, trauma
- Pregnancy, puerperium
- Long distance travel
- Use of combined oral contraceptives

Inherited
- Antithrombin deficiency
- Protein C deficiency
- Protein S deficiency
- Factor V Leiden (activated protein C resistance, APCR)
- Prothrombin PT20210A allele

Acquired
- Antiphospholipid antibody, lupus anticoagulant
- Hyperhomocysteinaemia
- Malignancy
- Myeloproliferative diseases

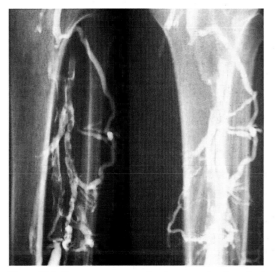

Figure 10.3 Contrast venogram showing extensive thrombosis with intraluminal filling defects and vessel occlusion

Box 10.3 Clinical features of familial thrombophilia
- Family history of venous thromboembolism
- First episode at early age
- Recurrent venous thromboembolism
- Unusual site of thrombosis—eg cerebral, mesenteric
- Thrombosis during pregnancy or puerperium
- Spontaneous venous thrombosis without environmental or acquired risk factor
- Recurrent superficial thrombophlebitis

Box 10.4 Recommended international normalised ratio ranges
2.0-3.0
- Treatment of deep vein thrombosis and pulmonary embolism
- Atrial fibrillation
- Mitral stenosis with embolism
- Transient ischaemic attack

3.0-4.5
- Recurrence of deep vein thrombosis or pulmonary embolism while taking warfarin
- Mechanical prosthetic heart valves

can either be primary or secondary to an underlying collagen vascular disorder. Laboratory diagnosis of this condition entails the detection of antibodies to cardiolipin or a lupus anticoagulant, or both. The latter causes in vitro a prolonged activated partial thromboplastin time and a prolonged dilute Russell's viper venom test, which corrects with excess phospholipids, but it is paradoxically associated in vivo with thrombosis. Lupus anticoagulants can also be induced by infections and drugs, and in these circumstances are not usually associated with thrombosis.

Anticoagulation

Warfarin
Warfarin is an oral anticoagulant that results in the synthesis by the liver of non-functional coagulation factors II, VII, IX, and X, as well as proteins C and S, by interfering with vitamin K metabolism.

Warfarin prolongs the prothrombin time, and dosage monitoring is achieved by a standardised form of this test, the international normalised ratio (INR).

Recommended target ranges and duration of treatment have been published; an INR target of 2.5 with a range of 2 to 3 being appropriate for most cases.

Warfarin treatment requires regular monitoring as over-treatment carries an important haemorrhagic risk, and warfarin requirements may be affected by intercurrent illness or concurrent drug treatment. Dental extraction or minor surgery is usually safe if the INR is less than 2.0, whereas for major surgery warfarin should be discontinued and parenteral heparin substituted.

In pregnancy warfarin is absolutely contraindicated from 6 to 12 weeks of gestation as it may damage the fetus. Because warfarin crosses the placenta and affects the fetus, heparin is increasingly being substituted throughout pregnancy as the drug of choice for thromboprophylaxis.

Reversal of a high INR can be addressed in several ways, depending on the circumstances. In the absence of bleeding, omitting warfarin is usually sufficient. Minor bleeding episodes can be treated with local measures and small doses of vitamin K. Life threatening bleeding requires resuscitation of the patient together with treatment with a prothrombin complex clotting factor concentrate; fresh frozen plasma can be used if concentrate is not available, but it is considerably less effective.

Heparin
Heparin is a parenterally active anticoagulant that acts by potentiating the antithrombotic effects of antithrombin and can be used for both prophylaxis and treatment of venous thromboembolic disease. Unfractionated heparin is usually given intravenously and is monitored by prolongation of the activated partial thromboplastin time. It has a narrow therapeutic range with complex pharmacokinetics and great interpatient variation in dose requirements. Low molecular weight heparins are replacing unfractionated heparin for the prophylaxis of medical and surgical patients and the treatment of venous thromboembolic disease. They can be administered by once daily subcutaneous injection without monitoring.

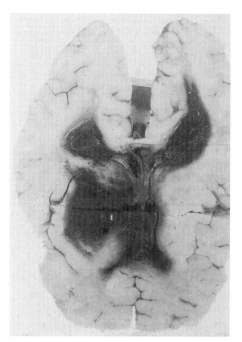

Figure 10.4 Intracerebral bleeding in patient taking warfarin

Table 10.5 Reversal of oral anticoagulation

Condition	Treatment
INR >4.5 without bleeding	Stop warfarin transiently and review
INR >4.5 with minor bleeding	Stop warfarin and consider small doses of intravenous vitamin K
Life threatening bleeding	Stop warfarin; give intravenous vitamin K 5 mg; give factors II, IX, X, and VII concentrate (50 units/kg factor IX) if available (if concentrate is unavailable give 15-25 ml/kg fresh frozen plasma)
Unexpected bleeding at any INR	Consider unsuspected underlying structural lesion

INR = international normalised ratio

Further reading
- Anon. Guidelines on oral anticoagulation: third edition. *Br J Haematol* 1998;101:374-87.
- Cattaneo M, Monzani ML, Martinelli I, Falcon CR, Mannucci PM. Interrelation of hyperhomocysteinemia, factor V Leiden, and risk of future venous thromboembolism. *Circulation* 1998;97:295-6.
- D'Angelo A, Selhub J. Homocysteine and thrombotic disease. *Blood* 1997;90:1-11.
- Dahlback B. Resistance to activated protein C as risk factor for thrombosis: molecular mechanisms, laboratory investigation, and clinical management. *Semin Hematol* 1997;34:217-34.
- Preston FE, Rosendaal FR, Walker ID *et al.* Increased fetal loss in women with heritable thrombophilia. *Lancet* 1996;348:913-16.
- Zivelin A, Griffin JH, Xu X *et al.* A single genetic origin for a common Caucasian risk factor for venous thrombosis. *Blood* 1997;89:397-402.

11 Malignant lymphomas and chronic lymphocytic leukaemia

G M Mead

The malignant lymphomas (non-Hodgkin's lymphoma and Hodgkin's disease) are a clinically and pathologically diverse group of cancers of largely unknown cause that are rapidly increasing in incidence. They are highly treatable and sometimes curable. Chronic lymphocytic leukaemia (CLL), the commonest adult leukaemia, shares many features with these cancers. The whole group constitutes about 5% of malignant diseases.

Pathology and staging

The non-Hodgkin's lymphomas (NHL) arise from malignant transformation of lymphocytes, deriving from B cells in about 85% of cases and T cells in most of the rest. Chronic lymphocytic leukaemia is largely a B cell malignancy. It has become increasingly clear that Reed Sternberg cells, which characterise Hodgkin's disease, are usually also of B cell origin.

Histopathologically, lymphomas comprise an admixture of identical (monoclonal) malignant cells with variable amounts of reactive lymphoid cells and stroma. The lymphomas are subcategorised by pathologists into about 20 different types on the basis of conventional cytological staining, special staining to determine subtype and lineage, and chromosomal abnormalities.

A diagnosis of lymphoma (or even B or T cell lymphoma) gives no clue to the natural course of the disease in an individual patient. Clinicians treating these patients take account of the histopathology and the history provided by the patient, as well as many other factors (for example, stage and age), before recommending treatment or advising about prognosis. The complexity of non-Hodgkin's lymphomas requires a simplified management approach, on the basis of division of cases into low grade (or indolent), intermediate, and high grade disease.

All patients with lymphoma or CLL require careful initial staging, usually comprising physical examination, measurement of an LDH level, computed tomography, and a bone marrow biopsy. Lymphomas are staged with the Ann Arbor system and CLL with the Binet system. Increasingly, treatment is decided on the basis of allocated stage together with an examination of other known prognostic factors. For NHL an International Prognostic Index (IPI) score is allocated which relates to prognosis.

Low grade non-Hodgkin's lymphomas and chronic lymphocytic leukaemia

The low grade non-Hodgkin's lymphomas and chronic lymphocytic leukaemia are rare in patients aged under 40 years and are predominantly diseases of elderly people (90% of patients are aged >50 years).

Nodal non-Hodgkin's lymphomas and chronic lymphocytic leukaemia

This group includes most of the follicular lymphomas and constitutes about 30% of the cases of non-Hodgkin's

---

> **Management of the malignant lymphoma is complex and is best carried out in specialised treatment centres**

> **Box 11.1 Ann Arbor staging system for lymphoma**
>
> **Site**
> - Stage I: Single lymphoid area or extranodal site (stage IE)
> - Stage II: Two lymphoid areas or extranodal sites on the same side of the diaphragm
> - Stage III: Lymphoid areas (including the spleen) on both sides of the diaphragm
> - Stage IV: Diffuse involvement of an extranodal organ(s) (liver, bone marrow)
>
> **Symptoms**
> - A: No symptoms
> - B: >10% weight loss, drenching night sweats, or unexplained fevers $\geqslant 38\,^{\circ}C$

> **Box 11.2 Binet staging system for chronic lymphocytic leukaemia**
>
> **Stage A** No anaemia or thrombocytopenia; fewer than three enlarged lymphoid areas
> **Stage B** As for stage A but three or more enlarged lymphoid areas
> **Stage C** Anaemia (concentration <100 g/l) and/or platelet count $<100 \times 10^9/l$

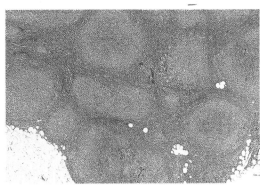

Figure 11.1 Follicular lymphoma (low power)

> **Box 11.3 Presenting features of low grade non-Hodgkin's lymphoma**
>
> - Painless peripheral lymphadenopathy
> - Abdominal mass (nodal or spleen)
> - Weight loss
> - Night sweats

> **Box 11.4 Presenting features of chronic lymphocytic leukaemia**
>
> - As for low grade non-Hodgkin's lymphoma
> - Asymptomatic: diagnosed coincidentally
> - Fatigue
> - Anaemia
> - Infection

lymphoma. Chronic lymphocytic leukaemia has a similar natural course. Diagnosis may be incidental (for example, from a routine blood count, as in CLL) or may follow a period of (often fluctuating) localised or generalised enlargement of lymph nodes or the spleen. These lymphomas are usually widespread at diagnosis, commonly (as in non-Hodgkin's lymphoma) or always (CLL) involving the bone marrow. Because of their indolent nature, however, there may be little or no initial effect on quality of life. Some patients, however, present with B symptoms or bulky widespread disease and need early treatment.

The management of these cancers is adjusted to their natural course. Cure can rarely be achieved, and the median overall survival in most series is 8-10 years. Prognosis relates to age (poorer when older) and particularly to the extent of disease judged in terms of bulk and effect of tumour. The outlook for chronic leukaemia worsens with increasing extent of disease at presentation and cytopenias (Binet stage B and C).

Patients who are well with non-threatening disease (eg low volume follicular lymphoma) may initially be watched without treatment—on occasions for many years. Initial treatment when needed generally comprises an alkylating agent-usually intermittent chlorambucil—with or without steroids for 4-6 months. This will often be highly successful in causing disease regression; relapse is, however, inevitable.

At relapse chlorambucil can be used again if initially effective, or, particularly for CLL, fludarabine, an antimetabolite can be given orally. Patients with follicular lymphoma often respond well at relapse to rituximab, a monoclonal B cell antibody given intravenously.

After several years the lymphomas may become refractory to treatment or may "transform" with change in histology and clinical course to an intermediate grade non-Hodgkin's lymphoma. If this occurs then combination chemotherapy is recommended, but the outlook is usually poor.

Newer treatment approaches under evaluation include (in younger patients) high dose chemotherapy with stem cell support, and for follicular lymphoma, monoclonal antibodies linked to a therapeutic radio-isotope (radio-immunotherapy).

Extranodal lymphoma (maltoma or marginal zone lymphoma)

These are indolent lymphomas that arise most commonly in the stomach, thyroid, parotid and lung—often evolving from a pre-existing inflammatory or autoimmune disease (for example, in the stomach gastritis relating to *Helicobacter pylori*, or in the parotid gland, Sjogren's syndrome). Gastric maltoma can be successfully managed in most cases by treatment of *H pylori* with appropriate antibiotics. Complete response, which is sustained, occurs in most cases—a unique example of regression of malignancy by treatment of infection. Remaining maltomas are generally managed with local radiotherapy with very high success rates.

The maltomas can progress to intermediate grade lymphomas. In addition, they can metastasise, usually to the other malt sites described above.

Intermediate grade non-Hodgkin's lymphoma

This is the most common grade of non-Hodgkin's lymphoma (65%) and affects any age group. It is rapidly increasing in incidence, although the reasons for this are uncertain.

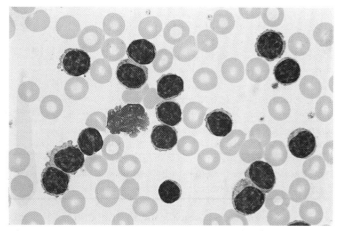

Figure 11.2 Peripheral blood film of patient with chronic lymphocytic leukaemia showing numerous malignant lymphocytes

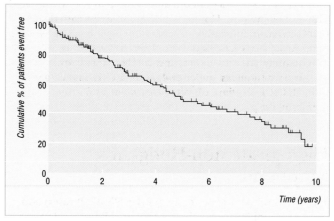

Figure 11.3 Survival curve of 160 patients with advanced follicular lymphoma: survival is prolonged, but there is no evidence of cure

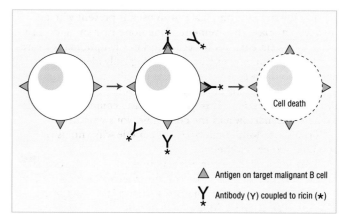

Figure 11.4 "Targeted" antibody therapy of lymphoma. The antibody delivers a toxin (ricin) to the lymphocytes bearing the appropriate surface antigen

Two-thirds of cases of this type of cancer arise within lymph nodes—patients present because of lymph node enlargement. The remaining cases may arise in almost any other tissue or organ (for example, gastrointestinal tract, skin, brain and bone), with symptoms appropriate to each site.

The most common type is diffuse large B cell lymphoma. These lymphomas occur at any age (median 65 years) and are rapidly progressive cancers that are often associated with B symptoms. Diagnosis and staging should be urgently performed then treatment with chemotherapy started. These cancers are curable in about 40% of cases. The prognosis relates to the patient's age, extent of spread, lactate dehydrogenase concentrations, and performance status.

The standard chemotherapy is a combination of cyclophosphamide, doxorubicin, vincristine, and prednisolone (CHOP), given intravenously at intervals of three weeks in the outpatient clinic on six occasions and sometimes supplemented by radiotherapy.

Relapse is not uncommon, and in the past it was associated with a poor outlook. However, younger patients with disease that has remained sensitive to chemotherapy may now be cured in up to 50% of cases using high dose chemotherapy. Survival in remaining patients is often measurable in months.

Newer treatments under evaluation are rituximab, given with CHOP at the time of initial treatment, and radio immunotherapy.

High grade non-Hodgkin's lymphoma

This grade of the disease is rare (under 5% of all cases) and comprises rapidly progressive cancers of children and young adults.

Lymphoblastic lymphoma is a T cell lymphoma identical to T cell acute lymphoblastic leukaemia, which occurs predominantly in young males who usually present with a mediastinal mass. Involvement of the bone marrow and central nervous system commonly occur. Burkitt's lymphoma is a rare B cell neoplasm of young adults, cytologically identical to B cell acute lymphoblastic leukaemia, that usually arises at extranodal sites, most commonly in the gastrointestinal tract—for example, the ileocaecal region. This lymphoma also commonly spreads to the bone marrow and the central nervous system.

Both these lymphoma types are curable with intensive combination chemotherapy.

Treatment of these cancers is urgent and may, if adequate precautions are not taken, be complicated by the acute tumour lysis syndrome resulting from breakdown of the lymphoma. This can lead to renal failure and possible death. Intrathecal chemotherapy to prevent relapse in the central nervous system is routinely used. Overall cure rates generally exceed 50%.

AIDS related non-Hodgkin's lymphoma

The immunosuppression associated with HIV infection has been associated with a noticeable increase in the incidence of non-Hodgkin's lymphoma and Hodgkin's disease.

These diseases arise in many cases because of uninhibited expansion of multiple clones of lymphocytes infected with Epstein-Barr virus. They are commonly high grade B cell neoplasms that arise at extranodal sites—for example, the brain and the ileocaecal area. The outlook for patients with these

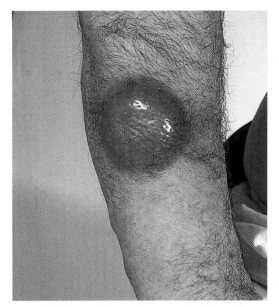

Figure 11.5 Intermediate grade non-Hodgkin's lymphoma arising in skin

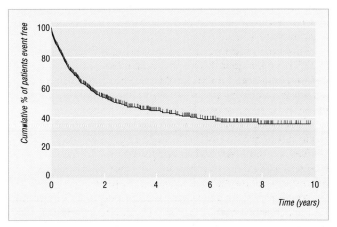

Figure 11.6 Survival of 760 patients with large cell non-Hodgkin's lymphoma (40% cure rate)

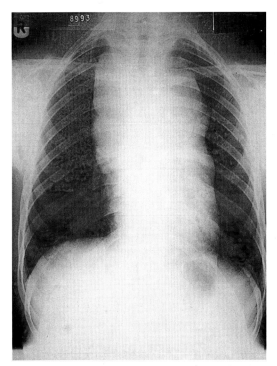

Figure 11.7 Anterior mediastinal mass in adolescent male: histological tests revealed lymphoblastic lymphoma

49

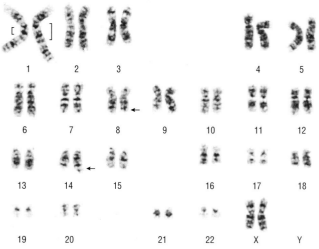

Figure 11.8 Karyotyping may aid lymphoma diagnosis. Here 8;14 translocation is shown in Burkitt's NHL

cancers has markedly improved since the introduction of effective antiretroviral therapy.

Hodgkin's disease

Pathology

Hodgkin's disease has classically been divided into four types. Recent studies suggest, however, that one type—lymphocyte predominant (LPHD)—is a clinically distinct B cell lymphoma often presenting with isolated enlargement of a peripheral lymph node.

The nodular sclerosing type constitutes 70-80% of cases of Hodgkin's disease and classically presents in young women with mediastinal and cervical nodal disease.

Mixed cellularity disease occurs predominantly in older males and is more commonly widespread. Lymphocyte depleted Hodgkin's disease is rare.

Clinical presentation and management

Hodgkin's disease most commonly presents as enlargement of supradiaphragmatic lymph nodes with or without B symptoms. Generalised pruritus can be a presenting feature in some cases. The spleen is involved in at least 30% of cases, and in the past the disease was detected with splenectomy. This procedure has now been abandoned as studies suggested no overall survival benefit from this procedure. Modern management relies on assessment of prognostic factors. The staging is as for non-Hodgkin's lymphoma with the Ann Arbor system.

Patients with stage I LPHD should be managed with localised irradiation with a high chance of cure. Increasingly, all other stage I or II cases are treated with a combined approach, receiving initial intravenous combination chemotherapy supplemented by irradiation with a high chance (95%) of cure. Patients with more extensive or symptomatic disease are treated primarily with combination chemotherapy, sometimes supplemented by irradiation to bulky sites. The drug combination ABVD (doxorubicin, bleomycin, vinblastine, and dacarbazine) is accepted standard therapy, given intravenously every two weeks for six months. Approximately 70% of patients receiving this treatment, sometimes supplemented by irradiation to bulky sites, will be cured. Fertility is usually preserved.

If relapse occurs, the standard treatment approach is with high dose chemotherapy supported by peripheral blood stem cell infusion. Cure rates of approximately 50% are achieved with this treatment approach.

Long term studies have suggested that overall cure rates for Hodgkin's disease are stable at 70-80%, although it is hoped that some of the newer chemotherapy approaches may improve these figures. Increasingly patients with Hodgkin's disease resume an entirely normal life once treatment has been completed. A particular concern, however, is an increased incidence of breast cancer in female patients who have received mantle radiotherapy.

Table 11.1 Clinical features of Hodgkin's disease _vs_ non-Hodgkin's lymphoma

	Hodgkin's disease	Non-Hodgkin's lymphoma
Incidence	Stable	Increasing
Age	Median 29 years	Increasing incidence with age
Sites	Nodal; supradiaphragmatic	Nodal or extranodal; any site
Clinical features	Mediastinal mass; itching; alcohol induced pain	Nil specific
Prognosis	70-80% cure	Highly variable by type; most incurable

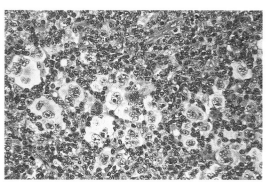

Figure 11.9 Reed Sternberg cells in a typical mixed inflammatory background characterise Hodgkin's disease

Further reading

- Harris NL, Jaffe ES, Stein H *et al.* A revised European-American classification of lymphoid neoplasms: a proposal from the International Lymphoma Study Group. *Blood* 1994;84:1361-92.
- International Non-Hodgkin's lymphoma prognostic factors project. Predictive model for aggressive non-Hodgkin's lymphoma. *N Engl J Med* 1993;329:987-94.
- Horning SJ. Natural history of and therapy for the indolent non-Hodgkin's lymphoma. *Semin Oncol* 1993;20:75-88.
- Dighiero G, Maloum K, Desablens B *et al.* Chlorambucil in indolent chronic lymphocytic leukaemia. *N Engl J Med* 1998;338:1506-14.
- Multani PS, Grossbard ML. Monoclonal antibody based therapies for hematologic malignancies. *J Clin Oncol* 1998;16:3691-710.
- Zucca E, Bertoni F, Roggero E, Cavalli F. Gastric marginal zone B-cell lymphoma of MALT type. *Blood* 2000;1996:410-19.
- Fisher RI, Gaynor ER, Dahlberg S *et al.* Comparison of a standard regimen (CHOP) with three intensive chemotherapy regimens for advanced non-Hodgkin's lymphoma. *N Engl J Med* 1993;328:1002-6.
- Ratner L, Lee J, Tang S *et al.* Chemotherapy for human immunodeficiency virus-associated non-Hodgkin's lymphoma in combination with highly active antiretroviral therapy. *J Clin Oncol* 2001;19:2171-8.
- Canellos GP, Anderson JR, Propert KJ *et al.* Chemotherapy of advanced Hodgkin's disease with MOPP, ABVD, or MOPP alternating with ABVD. *N Engl J Med* 1992;327:1478-84.

Dr Dina Choudhury provided the blood film showing chronic lymphocytic leukaemia (Figure 11.2).

12   Blood and marrow stem cell transplantation

Andrew Duncombe

History

Experiments in the 1950s showed that haemopoiesis could be restored in irradiated animals by engraftment of transfused marrow. Attempts to translate this into clinical practice were hindered by immunological problems of transfer between individuals which we now recognise as rejection and graft versus host disease.

With further understanding of the human leucocyte antigen system, rapid clinical progress was made during the 1970s such that bone marrow transplantation soon became an established treatment for some immune deficiency and malignant diseases.

What is a stem cell transplant?

Transplantation is the reconstitution of the full haemopoietic system by transfer of the pluripotent cells present in the bone marrow (stem cells). This usually requires prior ablation of the patient's own marrow by intensive chemotherapy or chemoradiotherapy.

The most appropriate generic term for the procedure is haemopoietic stem cell transplantation, which may be subdivided according to the donor source and further subdivided into the site of stem cell procurement.

Allogeneic transplantation is when another individual acts as the donor—usually a sibling of the patient, sometimes a normal volunteer. All cases, however, require a full or near HLA match—that is, they should be HLA compatible. Autologous transplantation is when the patient acts as his or her own source of stem cells.

Originally, stem cells were procured from the bone marrow by direct puncture and aspiration of bone marrow and reinfused intravenously, a procedure known as bone marrow transplantation. Recently, it has been shown that stem cells derived from the bone marrow can be liberated into the peripheral blood, where the cells are harvested with a cell separation machine. Transplants with this stem cell material are known as peripheral blood stem cell transplants. Stem cells derived from the bone marrow or peripheral blood may be used in either an allogeneic or an autologous setting.

Allogeneic transplantation

Suitability
Owing to the profound toxicity of the transplant procedure, potential recipients should be otherwise healthy and usually aged <55 years. As bone marrow contains B and T lymphocytes along with macrophages the donor and recipient must be fully or near fully HLA matched to prevent life threatening graft versus host disease or rejection.

This restricts the availability of potential donors. Within the patient's family the greatest chance of a full HLA match is with a sibling. An average recipient in Western countries has about a 1 in 4 chance of having a sibling who is fully HLA matched.

With this restriction in allogeneic transplantation, interest has surrounded the use of normal volunteer donors who show a close HLA match to the potential recipient. This has been achieved by the establishment of bone marrow registries in

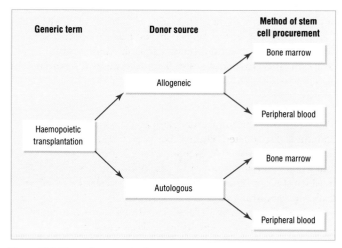

Figure 12.1 Transplant terminology

Table 12.1 Indications for allogeneic transplantation

Conditions for which it is the sole chance of cure
Primary immunodeficiency syndromes
Aplastic anaemia
Thalassaemia
Sickle cell disease
Inborn errors of metabolism
Chronic myeloid leukaemia
Myelodysplasia
Multiple myeloma

Conditions where there is probably benefit over conventional treatment
Acute myeloid leukaemia (first or second complete remission)
Acute lymphoblastic leukaemia(first or second complete remission)*

*In children, where acute lymphoblastic leukaemia (ALL) is the commonest leukaemia, the majority will be cured by standard chemotherapy alone without resort to transplantation, which is reserved for those who relapse.

which volunteers agree to donate marrow. There are three such registries in Britain—the British Bone Marrow Registry run by the National Blood Service, the Welsh Bone Marrow Donor Registry, run by the Welsh Blood Service, and the Anthony Nolan panels. There is also an international registry known as Bone Marrow Donors Worldwide.

Although the size of bone marrow registries is increasing, the heterogeneity of the HLA complex means that there is still a shortage of appropriately matched donors for all potential recipients.

Autologous transplantation

Suitability
Less immunological disturbance occurs in autologous than in allogeneic transplantation as the donor and the recipient are the same individual; the stresses on the cardiorespiratory, skin, and mucosal systems, however, are similar. Autologous recipients therefore should still be otherwise healthy but can be aged up to about 70 years.

Indications
The indications for autologous transplantation are being continuously evaluated by a number of studies, including randomised control trials, in many diseases, particularly malignancy. The indications can best be broken down into those in which there is now proved benefit in randomised controlled trials, those in which there is probable benefit, and those in which there is possible benefit. Results in solid tumours including RCTs in breast cancer have generally been disappointing.

Obtaining the graft

Bone marrow is harvested by puncture of the iliac crests under general anaesthesia. It is aspirated directly from the marrow cavity with marrow biopsy needles.

Up to a litre of marrow may be needed to provide sufficient stem cells for transplantation. The procedure is well tolerated, requiring only simple analgesia postoperatively. Serious complications are rare.

In peripheral blood stem cell transplantation, stem cells are mobilised into the blood by single agent chemotherapy or a haemopoietic growth factor (for example, granulocyte colony stimulating factor), or both. When the white blood count rises after 5-12 days, the individual is connected to a cell separation machine, blood is drawn off and spun in a centrifuge, and stem cells are harvested while the remaining blood elements are returned to the patient. The procedure takes 2-4 hours and is well tolerated.

Peripheral blood stem cell transplantation (PBSCT) is gradually replacing bone marrow transplantation as the

Box 12.1 Indications for autologous transplantation
- **Proven benefit in randomised controlled trials**
  Relapsed non-Hodgkin's lymphoma (intermediate and high grade)
  Acute myeloid leukaemia (first or second complete remission)
  Multiple myeloma
- **Probable benefit**
  Relapsed Hodgkin's disease
  Acute lymphoblastic leukaemia (first or second complete remission)
  Relapsed testis cancer
- **Possible benefit**
  Chronic myeloid leukaemia
  Severe autoimmune disease

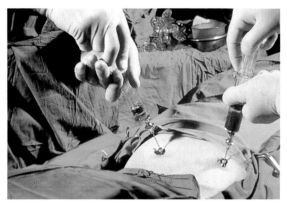
Figure 12.2 Haematologists performing bone marrow harvest

Box 12.2 Peripheral blood compared to bone marrow as source of haemopoietic stem cells
- **Advantages**
  Simple procedure: no general anaesthetic
  More rapid engraftment
  Cheaper
  ? Lower relapse rates in CML allografts
- **Disadvantages**
  ? Higher rates of chronic GvHD
  ? Lower survival rates in aplastic anaemia

No definitive answer yet to whether either source is superior

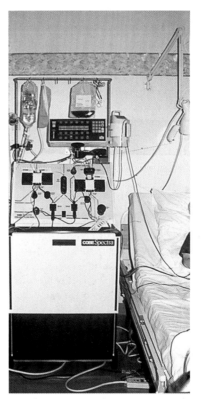
Figure 12.3 Extracorporeal cell separation device for collection of peripheral blood stem cells, showing inlet and outlet intravenous lines; collected stem cell product is in bag above machine

procedure of choice as no general anaesthesia is needed, engraftment is more rapid with earlier discharge from hospital, and the procedure is cheaper.

An alternative source of stem cells is umbilical cord blood which is gaining popularity as cord blood banks become established in the UK and Europe.

Transplantation procedures

Allogeneic transplantation

The recipient is treated with high dose chemotherapy or chemoradiotherapy to ablate the bone marrow (conditioning). On the day after the treatment has ended, bone marrow or peripheral blood stem cells are harvested from the donor, and the transplant is performed by infusing the stem cells intravenously. After a period of severe myelosuppression lasting 7-21 days, engraftment of the transplanted material takes place.

Autologous transplantation

The recipient, while in disease remission, undergoes a bone marrow or peripheral blood stem cell harvest. The stem cells are processed and frozen in liquid nitrogen. The recipient then starts conditioning. One day after the conditioning has ended, the stem cell product is thawed and infused intravenously. The bags are thawed rapidly by transfer directly from a liquid nitrogen container into water at 37-43 °C. The product is infused intravenously, rapidly through an indwelling central line. Myelosuppression and engraftment follow as described above.

One major procedural difference between allogeneic and autologous transplantation is the requirement for immunosuppression in allografts to prevent graft versus host disease and rejection. This is achieved with combinations of cyclosporin A and methotrexate or with in vitro or in vivo depletion of T cells using monoclonal antibodies.

Outcomes

Disease free survival rates continue to improve and depend on a number of factors. Key ones are shown in Table 12.2.

Sibling matched allograft: five year disease free survival rates for patients transplanted early in the disease are shown below

Thalassaemia	90%
Chronic myeloid leukaemia	65%
Acute leukaemia	55%
Myelodysplasia	55%

Autograft: five year event free survival rates are shown below

Responsive relapsed non-Hodgkin's lymphoma	50%
Myeloma	25%
Relapsed testis cancer	30%

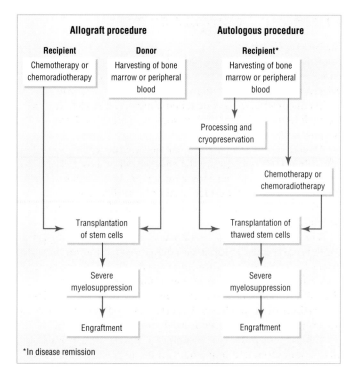

Figure 12.4 Transplantation procedures

Table 12.2 Factors affecting long term survival

Factor	Better outcome with:
Transplant type	Sibling allo. > Unrelated allo. > Autologous
Recipient age	Younger patients
Disease status	Early in disease or first remission
Presence or absence of GvHD	GvHD survivors
Donor age	Younger donors
CMV serology	Donor and recipient negative

Box 12.4 Early complications of transplants

- **Chemoradiotherapy**
  Nausea and vomiting
  Reversible alopecia
  Fatigue
  Dry inflamed skin
  Mucositis
  Veno-occlusive disease
- **Infections**
  Bacterial (Gram negative and positive)
  Viral
    Herpes zoster
    Cytomegalovirus (particularly pneumonitis)
  Fungi
    Candida
    Aspergillus
  Atypical organisms
    Pneumocystis (PCP)
    Toxoplasma
    Mycoplasma
    Legionella
- **Acute GvHD (allograft only)**
  Rash
  Diarrhoea
  Jaundice

Procedural complications

Early complications

Allogeneic and autologous procedures are associated with considerable morbidity and mortality. Overall, transplant-related mortality for autologous recipients is 2-15%, for recipients of sibling HLA matched allografts it is 15-30%, and for recipients of allografts from volunteer, unrelated donors it is up to 40%.

Nausea and vomiting from chemoradiotherapy is controllable with drugs, but the widespread mucosal damage to the gastrointestinal tract causes mucositis, which can be more difficult to control. Oral ulceration, buccal desquamation, oesophagitis, gastritis, abdominal pain, and diarrhoea may all be features.

The severe myelosuppression after the transplant, together with immune dysfunction from delayed reconstitution or graft versus host disease, predisposes to a wide variety of potentially fatal infections with bacterial (Gram positive and negative), viral, fungal, and atypical organisms. Prophylactic antibiotics may reduce their incidence, but astute surveillance and prompt intervention with intravenous antibiotics are mandatory.

Infection with the herpes simplex virus or the herpes zoster virus is common, and infection with the herpes zoster virus in particular may present with fulminant extensive lesions.

The most feared viral infection after allografting, however, is caused by cytomegalovirus. This may give rise to fulminant cytomegalovirus pneumonitis, which still has a high mortality despite newer antiviral drugs.

Fungal infections with Candida species are common, and disseminated aspergillus infection is particularly serious. Preventive measures include the use of broad spectrum antifungal agents prophylactically and the use of air filtration in positive pressure isolation cubicles for patients throughout transplant.

Graft versus host disease is classified as acute if occurring within 100 days of transplantation and chronic if occurring after that time. Acute graft versus host disease ranges from a mild self limiting condition to a fatal disorder. The mainstay of treatment remains immunosuppression, but severe disease resistant to immunosuppressive therapy is usually fatal. Chronic graft versus host disease is associated with collagen deposition and sclerotic change in the skin, giving a wider distribution of affected organs than the acute disease. Treatment is with immunosuppression aimed at controlling disease and ameliorating symptoms.

Follow up treatment and surveillance

For allograft recipients, immunosuppression needs careful monitoring to avoid toxicity. Unlike transplant recipients of solid organs, recipients of haemopoietic transplants do not need lifelong immunosuppression, and cyclosporin is normally discontinued about six months after transplantation. Prophylactic prescription for specific infections is required, including penicillin to prevent pneumococcal sepsis secondary to hyposplenism, aciclovir to prevent reactivation of the herpes simplex virus and the herpes zoster virus, and cotrimoxazole or pentamidine to prevent infection with *Pneumocystis carinii*.

Regular haematological follow up is mandatory, and psychological support from the transplant team, family, and friends is vital for readjustment to normal life.

Despite all the above potential complications, most patients return to an active, working life without ongoing treatment.

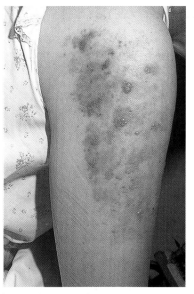

Figure 12.5 Severe herpes zoster on upper arm after transplant

Box 12.5 Clinical features of graft versus host disease

- **Acute**
  Skin rash (typically palms and soles)
  Abdominal pain
  Profuse diarrhoea
  Jaundice (intrahepatic cholestasis)
- **Chronic**
  Sclerotic atrophic skin
  Sicca syndrome
  Mucosal ulceration
  Malabsorption syndromes
  Recurrent chest infections
  Cholestatic jaundice
  Joint movement restriction
  Hyposplenic infections, e.g. Pneumococcus
  Myelosuppression

Table 12.3 New therapeutic agents in graft versus host disease

Agent type	Mode of action
Campath 1H	Anti-lymphocyte monoclonal antibody—destroys T cells in vivo
FK506	Powerful T cell function suppressor
Mycophenolate mofetil	Inhibits T cell function
Extracorporeal photopheresis	UV inactivation of GvHD-inducing lymphocytes

Box 12.6 Late complications of transplantation

- Infertility (both sexes)
- Hypothyroidism
- Secondary malignancy
- Late sepsis due to hyposplenism
- Cataracts (secondary to total body irradiation)
- Psychological disturbance

Box 12.7 Low intensity *v* standard intensity conditioning protocols

- Lower immediate toxicity
- ? Lower transplant related mortality overall
- ? Higher risk of relapse
- Long term survival comparisons awaited

Recent advances

Our capability to measure miniscule amounts of residual disease after transplant by polymerase chain reaction (PCR) methodology has enabled trials of therapy to prevent emerging relapse by the use of infusions of lymphocytes from the donor (DLI). Careful scheduling and dosing has treated post-allograft molecular relapse in CML patients and may be applicable to other malignancies.

The use of lower intensity conditioning protocols in allograft recipients (sometimes called mini-allos) may reduce toxicity and extend the indications and age range for allografts.

The future

Haemopoietic transplantation is an exciting and rapidly developing field. The molecular revolution has already resulted in greatly improved DNA matching at the HLA gene loci, which should ensure that transplants from volunteer unrelated donors will be more widely applicable and more successful. The haemopoietic stem cell's property of infinite self renewal makes it an ideal target vehicle for insertion of genes. Candidates include factor VIII gene replacement in haemophilia.

Recent discoveries in the ability of haemopoietic stem cells to change into cells of many unrelated tissues such as heart, brain, liver, and skin has raised the possibility of using them as a resource to repair failing organs. Although early embryo cells show the greatest plasticity, even stem cells from adults retain some ability to differentiate into other human tissues.

The future therapeutic potential of haemopoietic stem cells is enormous, but many clinical challenges remain. The next decade is likely to see major advances in haemopoietic stem cell therapies.

Box 12.8 Future developments in haemopoietic transplantation

- Improved DNA matching techniques for volunteer unrelated donors
- Umbilical cord blood banks to expand to provide source of autologus stem cells as "spare parts" for future failing organs
- Haemopoietic stem cells to repair cardiac muscle damage from myocardial infarcts
- Gene therapy
  Haemophilia
  Haemoglobinopathy
  Cystic fibrosis

Further reading
- Atkinson K. *Clinical bone marrow transplantation*. Cambridge: Cambridge University Press, 2000.
- Atkinson K. *The BMT data book*. Cambridge: Cambridge University Press, 1997.
- Forman SJ, Blume KG, Donnall TE. *Haemopoietic cell transplantation*. Blackwell: Oxford, 1998.
- Treleaven J, Barrett J. *Bone marrow transplantation in practice*. Edinburgh: Churchill Livingstone, 1992.

I am grateful to Dr J Treleaven and Mr R Smith for providing photographic material.

13 Haematological disorders at the extremes of life

Adrian C Newland, Tyrrell G J R Evans

Infants

Anaemia in neonates

The haemoglobin concentration at birth is 159-191 g/l. It rises transiently in the first 24 hours but then slowly falls to as low as 95 g/l by nine weeks. By six months, the concentration stabilises at around 125 g/l, the lower end of the adult range, increasing towards adolescence. The normal fall in haemoglobin concentration seen in full term infants is accentuated in prematurity and may fall to less than 90 g/l by four weeks. Preterm infants are particularly prone to multiple nutritional deficiencies because of rapid growth. Pronounced anaemia may be assumed if the infant gains insufficient weight or is fatigued while feeding.

Haemolytic disease in newborn infants

Haemolytic disease in newborn infants is due to destruction of fetal red cells by antibodies from the mother that cross the placenta. The most important are antibodies to the RhD antigen. Maternal immunisation is preventable by the prophylactic use of anti-D immunoglobulin, and since its introduction in the 1960s the number of affected babies has fallen dramatically. Anti-D immunoglobulin is administered to non-sensitised RhD negative women, but prophylaxis may fail.

In severely affected fetuses, mortality used to be as high as 40%, with only exchange transfusion available after delivery to correct anaemia and prevent kernicterus. Intrauterine transfusion, initially via the intraperitoneal route, was introduced to prevent problems in the fetus. However, it was the development in the early 1980s of intravascular blood transfusion using fetoscopy into the umbilical artery that dramatically improved survival. Hydrops can be readily reversed in utero, and even in the most severe group the survival rate has been 85%.

Anaemia associated with infection

Cytomegalovirus, rubella, toxoplasmosis, and more rarely congenital syphilis may be associated with anaemia, due either to haemolysis or to bone marrow suppression. More recently, human parvovirus B19 has been identified as a cause of anaemia and fetal damage. In early pregnancy maternal infection may lead to spontaneous abortion, but in later pregnancy it may lead to selective depression of erythropoiesis with profound anaemia and the development of hydrops. It may also induce an aplastic crisis or chronic haemolysis in normal children but is a major problem in those with an underlying haemoglobinopathy.

Malaria is a major health hazard worldwide, and easier travel to endemic areas has increased the problem. Inadequate or non-existent prophylaxis has led to an increase in cases over the past few years; unsuspected infection in neonates, usually caught from the mother, may be associated with a high mortality.

The haemoglobinopathies

β Thalassaemia major is an inherited haemoglobin disorder caused by reduction in β globin chain synthesis. It affects primarily people from the Indian subcontinent and of Mediterranean origin. It presents during the first year of life after the switch from fetal to adult haemoglobin. If production of the latter is reduced, anaemia occurs. The infant presents

---

Box 13.1 Common causes of anaemia in newborn infants

- **Blood loss:**—occult bleeding (fetomaternal, fetoplacental, twin to twin); obstetric accidents; internal bleeding; iatrogenic
- **Increased destruction:**—immune haemolytic anaemia; infection; haemoglobinopathies; enzymopathies
- **Decreased production:**—infection; nutritional deficiencies

---

Table 13.1 Normal haematology values in newborn infants

	Hb (g/l)	RBC ($\times 10^{12}$/l)	MCV (fl)	Nucl. RBC (per ml)
Day 1	168-212	4.44-5.84	109.6-128.4	500
Week 1	150-196	4.0-5.6	93.0-131.0	0
Week 4	111-143	3.2-4.0	92.9-109.1	0
Week 8	98-116	2.9-3.9	105.0-81.0	0
Week 12	104-122	3.4-4.0	80.1-95.9	0

Hb, haemoglobin; RBC, red blood cells; MCV, mean cell volume; Nucl., nucleated

---

Box 13.2 Haemolytic disease in newborn infants

Recommendations for prophylactic anti-D immunoglobulin in RhD negative women
- After delivery if the infant is Rh positive
- After abortion (therapeutic or spontaneous)
- To cover antenatal procedures (amniocentesis, chorionic villus sampling)
- After threatened abortion or miscarriage
- Antenatally at 28 and 34 weeks (not yet universal)

Reasons for failure of prophylaxis
- Failure of administration (commonest cause)
- Inadequate dosage (routine Kleihauer tests should be performed)
- Earlier sensitisation that may not be detectable at birth
- Poor injection technique (should be deep intramuscular)

Box 13.3 HIV infection

- HIV may produce a chronic multisystem disease in children
- Perinatal transmission of the virus from an infected woman is the primary route of exposure to the fetus (20-40% of pregnancies)
- Thrombocytopenia occurs in up to 15% of children with HIV infection
- Anaemia is also common, occurring early, usually with the normocytic, normochromic features of chronic disease
- Leucopenia and lymphopenia are also seen, in which the bone marrow shows non-specific features of chronic infection

with failure to thrive, poor weight gain, feeding problems, and irritability. The blood appearances are typical, with severe anaemia associated with microcytosis and hypochromia with pronounced morphological change in the red cells. The infant will be dependent on transfusions unless bone marrow transplantation is feasible. The carrier state (thalassaemia minor or thalassaemia trait) mimics iron deficiency, from which it must be differentiated.

β Thalassaemia presents a similar picture, and the condition is a common cause of stillbirth in South East Asia.

Sickle cell disease

Sickle cell disease is caused by a structural abnormality of the β chain and is associated with a steady state haemoglobin of 50-110 g/l. In homozygous sickle cell disease the haemoglobin forms crystals, distorting the red blood cells into a rigid sickle cell shape. It is these sickle cells that block the microvasculature, causing sickle cell crises. Mortality and morbidity are increased at all ages, with the peak incidence of death at age 1-3 years. Sickle cell crises are precipitated by infection, hypoxia, dehydration, cold, and exhaustion and are particularly common in adverse environmental or poor socioeconomic conditions. In infants, crises present with the clinical problems of infection, splenic sequestration, and dactylitis. Towards the end of the first year, painful vaso-occlusive crises are more common, and pneumococcal septicaemia related to splenic dysfunction is particularly apparent.

Genetic counselling and prenatal diagnosis have made an important contribution to reducing the number of affected children in countries with a comprehensive screening programme.

Disorders of haemostasis

Deficiencies of clotting factor VIII (haemophilia A) or factor IX (haemophilia B or Christmas disease) may present symptomatically in the first days of life, with spontaneous bleeding. Bleeding from the cord or intracranial haemorrhage, however, are fortunately rare. Severe bleeding usually occurs at, for example, circumcision or when mobility increases. Both disorders of coagulation affect 1 in 10 000 of the population. They are X linked and clinically indistinguishable. The diagnosis may be suspected from the family history and can be confirmed antenatally.

Thrombocytopenia

Healthy infants have a platelet count in the adult range ($150-400 \times 10^9/l$). Thrombocytopenia is the most common haemostatic abnormality in newborn infants, occurring in up to a quarter of babies admitted to neonatal intensive treatment units. Asphyxia at birth, infection, and disseminated intravascular coagulation are the most common causes of thrombocytopenia. It may also occur after exchange transfusion. Platelet transfusions should be given to any infant whose count is $<20\ 10^9/l$.

Maternal autoimmune thrombocytopenia may be associated with neonatal thrombocytopenia because of placental transfer of antiplatelet antibodies. Fetal platelet counts rarely drop below $50 \times 10^9/l$, and intracranial haemorrhage is rare either prenatally or at birth. However, the count may fall in the first few days of life, and treatment may be needed at this stage.

There are no reliable predictors of severe thrombocytopenia. Treatment includes platelet transfusions and corticosteroids, but intravenous immunoglobulin is safe and effective in over 80% of infants.

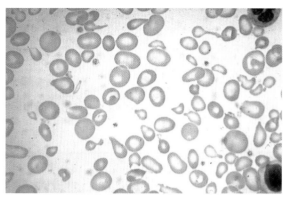

Figure 13.1 Peripheral blood of patient with Hb H disease showing pale red cells (hypochromia) with variation in size and shape (anisopoikilocytosis)

Table 13.2 Features of α thalassaemia

Syndrome	Haematological abnormalities	Diagnosis
Silent carrier (-α/αα)*	No anaemia or microcytosis	1-2% Hb Bart's[†]
Thalassaemia trait (-α/-α)	Mild anaemia and microcytosis	3-10% Hb Bart's
Hb H disease (-/-α)	Moderate microcytic, hypochromic haemolytic anaemia	20-40% Hb Bart's
Hb Bart's hydrops syndrome (--/--)	Severe microcytic hypochromic anaemia (lethal)	80% Hb Bart's, 20% Hb H[‡]

*Where αα/αα is normal (that is, 4 α genes) and -α represents deletion of one α gene on a chromosome
[†]Bart's γ$_4$ tetramers
[‡]Hb H β$_4$ tetramers

Antenatal screening for carrier detection of sickle cell disease (with subsequent study of the partners of positive women) should be carried out so that prenatal diagnosis can be offered

In up to 30% of all new cases patients will have no family history of coagulation disorders, and such cases are therefore new mutations

Box 13.4 Common causes of thrombocytopenia

- Immune mediated
    Neonatal alloimmune thrombocytopenia
    Maternal immune thrombocytopenia purpura
    Drug-induced
- Infection
    Viral—eg cytomegalovirus, HIV, rubella
    Toxoplasmosis
- Post exchange transfusion
- Disorders of haemostasis
    Disseminated intravascular coagulation
    Maternal pre-eclampsia
    Rhesus isoimmunisation
    Hypothermia, hypoxia
    Type IIB von Willebrand's disease
- Liver disease
- Giant haemangioma
- Hereditary thrombocytopenia
- Marrow infiltration

Neonatal alloimmune thrombocytopenia is associated with severe thrombocytopenia, and intracranial haemorrhage is seen in up to 15% of infants. Maternal platelet counts are normal, and maternal alloantibodies are directed against paternally derived antigens on the infant's platelets (usually HPA-1). In at risk pregnancies fetal blood sampling by cordocentesis should be used to confirm the HPA-1 status. Treatment relies on platelet transfusions in utero, but high dose intravenous immunoglobulin may be of some benefit.

Vitamin K deficiency
Haemorrhagic disease in newborn infants may be associated with vitamin K deficiency. It may be seen in otherwise healthy term infants, especially if they are being breast fed. The deficiency may be precipitated if the mother is taking anticonvulsant drugs or warfarin. It may present soon after birth with generalised bruising and internal bleeding, or as late as age one month.

Treatment is now aimed at prevention by administering vitamin K prophylaxis, although some controversy remains about whether this should be given orally or parenterally.

Elderly people

Haemoglobin concentration gradually declines from the age 60 years, with a more rapid fall over the age of 70. The fall is accompanied, however, by a widening of the reference range, such that age dependent ranges are of little value in individuals.

Concentration should be considered in association with the clinical history. In older patients the lower end of the normal range should be reduced to 110 g/l.

Iron deficiency anaemias
Between 10 and 20% of elderly people will be anaemic, usually with iron deficiency. In many this will be nutritional, owing to difficulties in obtaining and eating food, for both medical and social reasons. The possibility of an occult gastrointestinal malignancy (for example, caecal carcinoma) leading to iron deficiency anaemia should be considered. Aspirin or non-steroidal anti-inflammatory drugs leading to occult gastrointestinal blood loss may also contribute. The problem may also be exacerbated in elderly people as gastric atrophy may occur, leading to poor absorption of iron supplements.

Box 13.5 Clinical associations in iron deficiency

Symptoms: lethargy, lassitude, reduced activity; shortness of breath; angina on effort; intermittent claudication
Signs: pallor, peripheral oedema; brittle nails, koilonychia; glossitis; stomatitis
Other gastrointestinal findings: oesophageal web; atrophic gastritis; subtotal villous atrophy with malabsorption

---

Oral supplements are usually well tolerated. They should be continued for three months after the haemoglobin concentration has returned to normal, to replenish the iron stores.

Megaloblastic anaemia
Folic acid deficiency also occurs readily in those who eat poorly and can be easily corrected by supplements. Pernicious anaemia due to vitamin B_{12} deficiency also occurs in middle and later life and may be associated with weakness and loss of sensation. Vitamin B_{12} stores normally fall in older people, and

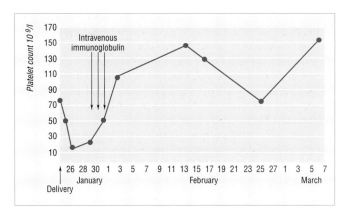

Figure 13.2 Response of neonate to intravenous immunoglobulin with thrombocytopenia secondary to maternal immune thrombocytopenic purpura. Copyright © 1984 Massachusetts Medical Society. All rights reserved.

Table 13.3 Haemorrhagic disease of newborn infants

Type	Clinical signs	Causes
Early (within 24 hours)	Severe bleeding, often internal	Mother receiving drugs affecting vitamin K—eg anticonvulsant (phenytoin), warfarin, antituberculosis drugs (rifampicin, isoniazid)
Classic (2-5 days)	Bruising or bleeding from gastrointestinal tract or after circumcision	Breast feeding, full term
Delayed (up to 1 month)	Intracranial haemorrhage, common	Prolonged breast feeding without prophylaxis; chronic diarrhoea, malabsorption, or oral antibiotics

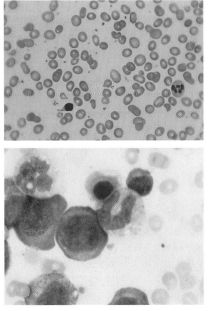

Figure 13.3 Megaloblastic anaemia: peripheral blood (top) showing macrocytes, tear drops, and multisegmented neutrophils; megaloblastic bone marrow (bottom) showing megaloblasts, giant metamyelocytes, and hypersegmented neutrophil

deficiency should always be considered with those developing dementia.

Care must be taken to differentiate megaloblastic anaemia from myelodysplastic syndrome, which may be associated with a refractory macrocytic anaemia. Serum concentrations of vitamin B_{12}, folate, and red cell folate should be measured, and occasionally a bone marrow examination may be indicated.

The importance of identifying any deficiency anaemia is that, although the effects may be relatively mild initially, they can progress and severely incapacitate a previously active elderly person. The deficiencies can be easily reversed, and supplements should be continued for as long as the underlying problem remains.

Anaemia of chronic disease

Any prolonged illness such as infection, malignant disease, renal disease, or connective tissue disorder may be accompanied by a moderate fall in the haemoglobin concentration. This seldom drops below 90-100 g/l, and it is typically normocytic and normochromic. Haematinics will not increase the haemoglobin concentration, which may improve only after treatment of the underlying condition. This condition may not always be apparent, and a general screen may be needed for underlying malignancy or systemic disease.

Malignancies

Most forms of malignancy are more common in elderly people than in the rest of the population. The myelodysplastic syndromes and chronic lymphocytic leukaemia are frequently found incidentally, and their diagnosis does not necessarily indicate the need for treatment. Each patient must be considered individually so that the possible benefits of treatment can be balanced against side effects and considered in the light of any improvement in the quality of life.

Further reading
- Hann IM, Gibson BES, Letsky EA, eds. *Fetal and neonatal haematology*. London: Baillière Tindall, 1991.
- Lilleyman JS, Hann IM, eds. *Pediatric hematology*. New York: Churchill Livingstone, 1992.
- Spiers ASD. Management of the chronic leukemias: special considerations in the elderly patient. Part 1. Chronic lymphocytic leukemias. *Hematology* 2001;6:291-314.

Box 13.6 Findings in anaemia of chronic disease

- Mild normocytic or microcytic anaemia
- Low serum iron concentration and iron binding capacity
- Reduced transferrin saturation
- Normal or raised serum ferritin concentration
- Increased iron in reticuloendothelial stores—eg bone marrow
- Defective iron transfer to red cell precursors
- Iron reduced in red cell precursors
- Increased red cell protoporphyrin

Box 13.7 Screening tests in anaemia of chronic disease[*]

- Review of peripheral blood film
- Erythrocyte sedimentation rate
- Liver and renal screen
- Chest radiograph
- Autoantibody screen
- Urine analysis
- Thyroid function studies
- Tumour markers
    Immunoglobulins (myeloma)
    Prostate specific antigen
    α Fetoprotein (liver)
    Carcinoembryonic antigen (gastrointestinal)

* After history and clinical examination.

Figure 13.2 is adapted with permission from Newland *et al.* (*N Engl J Med* 1984;310:261-2).

14   Haematological emergencies

Drew Provan

Patients with both malignant and non-malignant haematological disease may present with dramatic and often life threatening complications of their diseases. General physicians must be able to recognise and start basic treatment, which may be life saving, in patients presenting with haematological emergencies.

This chapter deals with five of the most common emergencies encountered by haematologists. Although none of these conditions is seen often in day to day clinical practice, recognition of the underlying disease processes is important in determining the likely cause of the abnormalities and is helpful in determining the specific treatment needed.

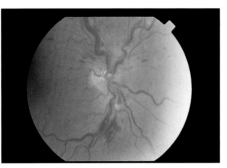

Figure 14.1 Fundal changes in patient with hyperviscosity (newly diagnosed myeloma with IgA concentration 50 g/l)

Hyperviscosity syndrome

This may be caused by several haematological conditions. Blood viscosity is a function of the concentration and composition of its components. A marked increase in plasma proteins (for example, monoclonal immunoglobulin in myeloma) or cellular constituents (for example, white blood cells in acute leukaemia) will raise the overall blood viscosity. This leads to sludging of the microcirculation and a variety of clinical manifestations. Hyperviscosity may present insidiously or acutely with neurological symptoms and signs.

Blood viscosity will often be more than four times the normal viscosity before symptoms occur. Patients with chronic disorders such as polycythaemia and myeloma are often physiologically well compensated for the degree of hyperviscosity and may complain only of mild headaches. In contrast, patients with acute leukaemia and a high white cell count may present in extremis; they become hypoxic from pulmonary involvement and are often obtunded, with a variety of neurological signs. Prompt treatment is needed to prevent permanent deficits. Elderly patients with impaired left ventricular function may experience decompensation due to their hyperviscosity, resulting in increasing congestive cardiac failure.

The definitive treatment of patients with hyperviscosity is dependent on the underlying pathology. For patients presenting with acute leukaemia, vigorous intravenous hydration and intensive chemotherapy often results in a rapid reduction in the white cell count. Leukapheresis may be used as an interim measure until chemotherapy exerts its full effect. For patients with myeloma or Waldenström's macroglobulinaemia (a low grade lymphoma characterised by production of monoclonal IgM, most of which is intravascular) plasmapheresis effectively reduces the paraprotein concentration. Plasmapheresis is more effective in reducing the level of IgM than IgG paraprotein since the former is predominantly intravascular while IgG is mainly extravascular.

> **Box 14.1 Causes of hyperviscosity**
> - Myeloma (especially IgA)
> - Waldenström's macroglobulinaemia (IgM paraprotein)
> - Polycythaemia
> - High white cell count (hyperleucocytosis)

> **Box 14.2 Symptoms and signs of hyperviscosity**
> - Mild headache
> - Neurological disturbance
>   Ataxia
>   Nystagmus
>   Vertigo
>   Confusion
>   Changes in mental state
>   Coma
> - Visual disturbance
>   Blurring of vision
>   Dilatation and segmentation of retinal veins
>   "Sausage" appearance of retinal veins
>   Risk of central retinal vein occlusion
> - Genitourinary or gastrointestinal bleeding

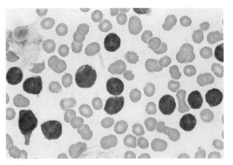

Figure 14.2 Blood film in patient with hyperviscosity due to hyperleucocytosis (4 year old child with newly diagnosed acute lymphoblastic leukaemia; white cell count 200×10^9/l)

> **Plasmapheresis may be used both for acute attacks and long term—for example, as palliative treatment for patients resistant to, or unable to tolerate, chemotherapy**

Sickle cell crisis

The sickling disorders (Hb SS, Hb SC, Hb S/β thalassaemia, and Hb SD) are inherited structural haemoglobin variants. Homozygous Hb SS in particular is associated with several complications, including recurrent vaso-occlusive crises, leg ulcers, renal impairment, hyposplenism, and retinopathy.

Box 14.3 Sickle cell crises

- **Vaso-occlusive:** In any tissue but especially bones, chest, and abdomen (eg splenic infracts); in cerebral vessels, leading to stroke
- **Aplastic:** In parvovirus B19 infection
- **Sequestration:** Particularly in infants and young children; massive pooling of red cells in spleen and other organs, leading to precipitous drop in haemoglobin
- **Haemolytic:** Further reduction in life span of red cells, leading to worsening anaemia and features of haemolysis
- **Chest syndrome:** Pleuritic pain and fever may mimic pneumonia or pulmonary embolism; progressive respiratory failure

Sickle cell crises include vaso-occlusive, aplastic, sequestration, and haemolytic episodes. The chest syndrome and the girdle syndrome are more severe forms of crisis associated with higher morbidity and mortality.

Crises may be precipitated by dehydration or infection; in many cases no obvious precipitant is found.

The aim of treatment is to break the vicious cycle of sickling: sickling results in hypoxia and acidosis, which in turn precipitate further sickling. This is exacerbated by dehydration, and a high fluid intake (70 ml/kg/24 h) is the cornerstone of management.

Also imperative in managing sickle cell crises is adequate pain relief—opiates, by continuous subcutaneous or intravenous infusions, may be needed. Arterial blood gas pressures should be performed and oxygen therapy prescribed if hypoxia is confirmed. It should be remembered that sickle cell patients are functionally asplenic and that infection is a common precipitant of crises. Broad spectrum antibiotics should be started while waiting for the results of blood and urine cultures.

It is important to recognise the patients who need urgent exchange transfusion to reduce the level of Hb S to below 30%. Transfusion should be started promptly if the patient has a severe chest syndrome (with pronounced hypoxia), has had a cardiovascular accident, or has priapism.

Spinal cord compression

Some patients may present at the haematology clinic with metastatic tumour deposits—for example, lymphoma or plasmacytoma—resulting in cord compression. Commonly, overt cord compression is preceded by signs consistent with root compression, with pain in the affected dermatome. Most patients with cord compression complain of pain—it is often constant and easily confused with that of pain due to degenerative disease. Often it is not until more overt neurological signs are manifested that a diagnosis of cord compression is considered.

The neurological signs accompanying cord compression vary according to both the rapidity of development of compression and the area of cord affected. Acute lesions often result in hypotonia and weakness, whereas chronic lesions are more often associated with the classic upper motor neurone signs of hypertonia and hyper-reflexia. The associated sensory loss is defined by the site of the lesion, but hyperaesthesia may be seen in the dermatome at the level of the lesion. More lateral lesions may result in a dissociative sensory loss—that is, ipsilateral loss of joint position sense and proprioception with contralateral loss of pain and temperature. Bladder and bowel disturbances often occur late, with the exception of the cauda equina compression syndrome, in which they are an early feature.

If cord compression is suspected the patient should be investigated with plain spinal radiography, which may show

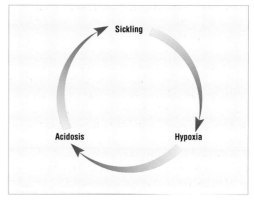

Figure 14.3 Vicious cycle in sickle cell crisis

Box 14.4 Treatment of sickle cell crises

- Vigorous intravenous hydration
- Adequate analgesia—for example, intravenous opiates
- Broad spectrum antibiotics
- Oxygen therapy
- Consider exchange blood transfusion

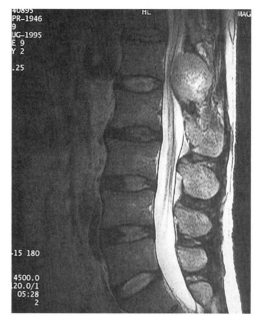

Figure 14.4 Magnetic resonance image showing spinal cord compression

Box 14.5 Symptoms and signs of cord compression

- Back pain
- Weakness in legs
- Upper motor neurone and sensory signs
- Loss of sphincter control (bowels/bladder)

Neurological advice should be obtained as in some cases surgical decompression may allow recovery of function

evidence of lytic lesions (as, for example, in myeloma). The definitive investigation is magnetic resonance imaging to delineate the level of the lesion and to help plan further treatment.

In a patient presenting de novo with cord compression further investigations (protein electrophoresis, measurement of prostatic specific antigen and other tumour markers, and chest radiography) are needed to elucidate the underlying cause. A formal biopsy of the lesion may be needed to determine the underlying condition.

In an acute presentation high dose dexamethasone (for example, 4 mg four times daily) is given. Further management depends on the underlying cause, but often a combination of chemotherapy and radiotherapy is given.

Disseminated intravascular coagulation

Disseminated intravascular coagulation describes the syndrome of widespread intravascular coagulation induced by blood procoagulants either introduced into or produced in the bloodstream. These coagulant proteins overcome the normal physiological anticoagulant mechanisms. The overall result, irrespective of cause, is widespread tissue ischaemia (due to clot formation, thrombi) and bleeding (due to consumption of clotting factors, platelets, and the production of breakdown products that further inhibit the coagulation pathway).

The diagnosis of disseminated intravascular coagulation is initially clinical and is confirmed by various blood tests. There are many causes of disseminated intravascular coagulation, including obstetric emergencies, infections, neoplasms, trauma, and vascular disorders.

Treatment is primarily directed at the underlying cause—for example, the use of antibiotics when infection is suspected, or removal of fetus and placenta with placental abruption or retained dead fetus syndrome. Disseminated intravascular coagulation generally resolves fairly quickly after removal of the underlying cause.

Interim supportive measures, such as intravenous hydration and oxygen therapy, are important. Correction of the coagulopathy entails the use of fresh frozen plasma, cryoprecipitate, and platelet transfusion. No uniform protocol exists for transfusing blood and blood products. Instead, for each patient the quantity of blood product used is decided after clinical evaluation and serial coagulation assays.

The use of intravenous heparin to treat disseminated intravascular coagulation remains controversial. Some evidence supports the value of heparin in the management of acute promyelocytic leukaemia, the dead fetus syndrome, and aortic aneurysm before resection. For other causes of disseminated intravascular coagulation the use of heparin is more uncertain and may actually worsen the bleeding.

Infection in patients with impaired immunity

Patients with a variety of haematological diseases are immunocompromised due to either their underlying disease or the treatment required for the condition. For example, patients with myeloma often present with recurrent infection as a result of the reduction in normal immunoglobulin concentrations associated with the paraproteinaemia. This susceptibility is compounded by the use of combination chemotherapy, which may render patients neutropenic.

Box 14.6 Causes of acute disseminated intravascular coagulation

- **Infection:** Especially Gram negative infections, endotoxic shock
- **Obstetric:** Placental abruption, intrauterine fetal death, severe pre-eclampsia or eclampsia, amniotic fluid embolism
- **Trauma:** Especially head injury, burns
- **Malignancy:** Carcinoma of prostate, lung, pancreas, ovary, and gastrointestinal tract
- **Miscellaneous:** Transfusion with incompatible blood group, drug reactions, hypothermia, venomous snake bite, transplant rejection
- **Vascular:** Aortic aneurysm, giant haemangioma

Box 14.7 Initial management of disseminated intravascular coagulation

- Treat as for severe bleeding/shock
- Establish intravenous access (large bore cannula)
- Restore circulating volume—with, for example, crystalloids
- Administer fresh frozen plasma and cryoprecipitate and regularly monitor full blood count, prothrombin time, and activated partial thromboplastin time
- Consider giving platelet transfusion
- Remove the underlying cause

Box 14.8 Clinical features of disseminated intravascular coagulation

Bleeding
- Spontaneous bruising
- Petechiae
- Prolonged bleeding from venepuncture sites, arterial lines, etc.
- Bleeding into gastrointestinal tract or lungs
- Secondary bleeding after surgery
- Coma (intracerebral bleeding)

Clotting
- Acute renal failure (ischaemia of renal cortex)
- Venous thromboembolism
- Skin necrosis or gangrene
- Liver failure (due to infection and hypotension)
- Coma (cerebral infarction)

Shock
- Due to underlying disease together with disseminated intravascular coagulation

Central nervous system
- Transient neurological symptoms and signs
- Coma
- Delirium

Lungs
- Transient hypoxaemia
- Pulmonary haemorrhage
- Adult respiratory distress syndrome

Table 14.1 Main investigations* for disseminated intravascular coagulation

Investigation	Positive result
Full blood count	Decreased platelet count
Prothrombin time	Increased
Activated partial thromboplastin time	Increased
Fibrinogen	Decreased
Fibrin degradation products/ D dimers	Increased

*Other investigations: urea and electrolytes, liver function tests, blood cultures, pulse oximetry (oxygen saturation)

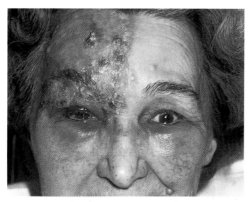

Figure 14.5 Herpes zoster virus affecting the ophthalmic division of the trigeminal nerve in patient with chronic lymphocytic leukaemia

> **Box 14.9 Risks of infection in patients with no spleen or hypofunctioning spleen**
>
> - With encapsulated organisms—for example, *Streptococcus pneumoniae* (60%), *Haemophilus influenzae* type b. *Neisseria meningitidis*
> - Less commonly—*Escherichia coli*, malaria, babesiosis, *Capnocytophaga canimorsus*

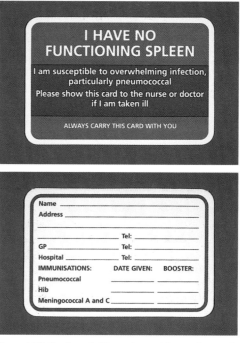

Figure 14.6 Card carried by patients with no spleen or hypofunctioning spleen

Several haematological disorders are now routinely treated in outpatient clinics with aggressive chemotherapy, so some patients in the community may be neutropenic as a result of this. Patients are educated to seek medical advice immediately if they develop any infection, since Gram negative septicaemia may lead rapidly to death. For patients receiving intensive chemotherapy presenting with fever while neutropenic, broad spectrum antibiotics should be started immediately. The choice of antibiotics depends on local microbiological advice in the light of the sensitivities of the micro-organisms in the region.

Patients with chronic lymphocytic leukaemia often have recurrent infection in the absence of neutropenia, because of the accompanying hypogammaglobulinaemia seen in this disorder. Frequent courses of antibiotics are often required. The role of regular intravenous immunoglobulin infusions to "boost" their immunity is debatable. Patients with chronic lymphocytic leukaemia may develop severe recurrent herpes zoster infections. Prompt treatment with aciclovir should always be given at the first suspicion of any herpetic lesions developing, and hospital referral for intravenous antibiotics and aciclovir should be considered if the lesions are not confined to a single dermatome or are in a delicate area—for example, ophthalmic division of the trigeminal nerve.

Patients who are functionally or anatomically asplenic are at high risk of infection with encapsulated organisms, especially *Streptococcus pneumoniae.*

Penicillin prophylaxis and immunisation reduces the incidence of these infections but does not abolish the risk completely. If any of these patients becomes acutely unwell the prompt administration of 1200 mg benzylpenicillin (if no history of allergy to penicillin) and prompt referral for further treatment may be life saving.

Dr Ken Tung, consultant radiologist, Southampton University Hospitals Trust, provided the magnetic resonance image in Figure 14.4. Figure 14.5, showing herpes zoster virus, is from *Clinical haematology—a postgraduate exam companion* by D Provan, A Amos and AG Smith. Reprinted by permission of Elsevier Science.

> **Box 14.10 Recommendations for patients with no spleen or hypofunctioning spleen***
>
> - Pneumococcal vaccine (Pneumovax II) 0.5 ml—two weeks before splenectomy or as soon as possible after splenectomy (for example, if emergency splenectomy is performed); reimmunise every 5-10 years
> - *H influenzae* type b (Hib) vaccine 0.5 ml
> - Meningococcal polysaccharide vaccine for *N meningitidis* type A and C 0.5 ml
> - Penicillin as prophylaxis (250 mg twice daily—for life)
>
> The three vaccines (subcutaneous or intramuscular) may be given at same time, but different sites should be used
> *Based on the guidelines for the prevention and treatment of infection in patients with an absent or dysfunctional spleen, *BMJ* 1996;312:430-4.

Further reading

- Beck JR, Quinn BM, Meier FA, Rawnsley HM. Hyperviscosity syndrome in paraproteinemia. Managed by plasma exchange; monitored by serum tests. *Transfusion* 1982;22(1):51-3.
- Davies SC, Oni L. Management of patients with sickle cell disease. *BMJ* 1997;315(7109):656-60.
- Gopal V, Bisno AL. Fulminant pneumococcal infections in "normal" asplenic hosts. *Arch Intern Med* 1977;137(11):1526-30.
- Working Party of the British Committee for Standards in Haematology Clinical Haematology Task Force. Guidelines for the prevention and treatment of infection in patients with an absent or dysfunctional spleen. *BMJ* 1996;312(7028):430-4.
- Levi M, ten Cate H, van der Poll T, van Deventer SJ. Pathogenesis of disseminated intravascular coagulation in sepsis. *JAMA* 1993;270(8):975-9.
- Torres J, Bisno AL. Hyposplenism and pneumococcemia. Visualization of *Diplococcus pneumoniae* in the peripheral blood smear. *Am J Med* 1973;55(6):851-5.
- Winkelstein A, Jordan PS. Immune deficiencies in chronic lymphocytic leukemia and multiple myeloma. *Clin Rev Allerg* 1992;10(1-2):39-58.

15   The future of haematology: the impact of molecular biology and gene therapy

Adele K Fielding, Stephen J Russell

This chapter will assess the impact of advances in science and technology on the practice of haematology and attempt to predict how haematology might change further over the next 10 to 15 years.

The major advances in scientific thought and technological development that have already changed the practice of modern haematology are likely to affect both laboratory diagnosis and treatment in the future. The first draft of the sequence of the human genome has now been published and "genomics" has mushroomed. The first clinical study in which gene therapy provided clear clinical benefit to patients has also been reported. Another very exciting development which may ultimately impact the practice of haematology is the discovery of the plasticity of post-natal stem cells. The identification of post-natal progenitor cells which can, ex vivo, be expanded and differentiated into many different cell types, may pave the way for treatment of genetic disorders of many kinds. While the debate about the ethical implications in the use of embryonic stem cells continues in many countries, post-natal stem cells may now offer a realistic and non-controversial alternative.

The chapter begins with an introduction to genomics and gene therapy, both of which are likely to have a role in most areas of haematological practice in the future. Three specific areas of haematology are then examined—haemoglobinopathy, haemophilia, and haematological malignancy—in each of which important innovations could be expected to change clinical practice.

Both diagnostically and therapeutically, the identification of the molecular pathology of the underlying disorder will continue to steer the future. The ability to make more accurate diagnoses in haematology is only just beginning to result in improved treatments. Careful clinical studies with well-designed correlative science that aims to ask and answer specific questions should remain the basis on which novel developments make their impact on routine practice.

Gene therapy

The term gene therapy is applied to any manoeuvre in which genes or genetically modified cells are introduced into a patient for therapeutic benefit. Gene therapy is still in its infancy, and despite the potential of the approach, clinical benefit has only recently been demonstrated.

Successful gene therapy depends on the availability of reliable methods for delivering a gene into the nuclei of selected target cells and subsequently ensuring the regulation of gene expression. Haematological cells are readily accessible for manipulation and so can be genetically modified outside the body and re-infused. The aim in the future, however, will be to modify the target cells without first removing them from the patient. Genes that are to be delivered to cells must first be inserted into plasmids. These small circular molecules of double stranded DNA derived from bacteria can then be used to transfer therapeutic genes to cells by physical methods or by insertion into recombinant viruses.

Whichever vector system is used, the barriers through which the therapeutic genes must be transported to reach their

---

Box 15.1 The future of haematology—diagnosis and treatment

Diagnosis
- Increasing automation giving quicker and more reliable results—eg automated cross matching; automated diagnostic polymerase chain reaction
- More DNA/RNA based diagnosis, allowing increased diagnostic precision—eg precise definition of genetic abnormalities; diagnosis with polymerase chain reaction
- More "near patient" testing, allowing rapid screening—eg haemoglobinometers, monitoring of anticoagulant treatment

Treatment
- New drugs—eg tailored to molecular abnormalities
- New biological agents—eg viruses and viral vectors, monoclonal antibodies
- Transplantation across tissue barriers—eg cord blood transplantation
- Blood substitutes—eg recombinant haemoglobin
- Gene therapy—probably for many haematological disorders

Table 15.1 Gene therapy strategies

Strategy	Potential application
Corrective replacement	Sickle cell disease—to replace the point mutation that causes the substitution of valine for glutamine on the sixth amino acid residue of the β globin chain
Corrective gene addition	Haemophilia—to introduce a gene for missing coagulation protein
Corrective antisense treatment	Low grade non-Hodgkin's lymphoma (NHL)—to introduce antisense oligonucleotides, preventing BCL2 overexpression, which is responsible for the failure of the lymphoma cells to undergo apoptosis
Pharmacological	Continuous production of interferon alfa, erythropoietin, or other therapeutic proteins
Cytotoxic	Leukaemia—targeted delivery of cytotoxic proteins
Prophylactic	Chemoprotection—drug resistance genes introduced into haemopoietic stem cells, conferring resistant phenotype, thus protecting against chemotherapeutic agents
Immunostimulatory	Idiotypic vaccination—in B cell tumours such as NHL and myeloma the variable region sequences of the surface immunoglobulin of the tumour cell provide a tumour specific antigen against which an individualised vaccine for each patient can be produced
Replicating virus therapy	Oncolytic viruses may be used to directly kill transformed cells

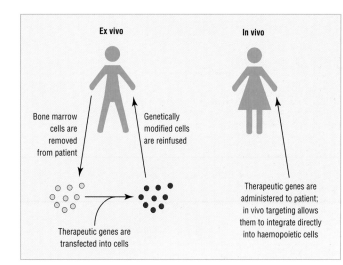

Figure 15.1 Ex vivo and in vivo gene transfer strategies

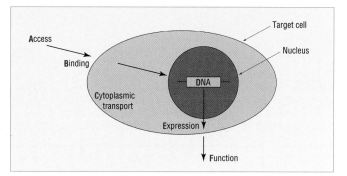

Figure 15.2 ABC of gene therapy—A vector must be able to access the cells to be transduced and bind and penetrate the membrane of the target cell. Once inside the nucleus, the exogenous DNA must be integrated into the cellular genome if stable expression is required. Gene expression must be at a high enough level and sufficiently regulated for clinical benefit

destination are the same. Many viral and non-viral vector systems are being developed to try to achieve the steps outlined here, and it is often difficult to choose the most appropriate vector for a particular application.

For gene therapy applications, where it is crucial to achieve gene expression in the progeny of the target (modified) cells, it is important to use a vector that stably inserts its genes into the chromosome of the host cell, and retrovirus vectors are the most suitable for this purpose. For direct in vivo gene delivery, vector attachment to a specific target cell is a vital additional requirement. Such vector targeting is at last beginning to look like a realistic possibility.

Genomics

Genomics can be defined as "the systematic study of all the genes of an organism". Recently, the number of genes in the human genome has been estimated at being between 30 000 and 40 000—many less than previously thought. The function of most of these genes currently remains unknown, although it is likely that this will not always be the case. It is now possible to obtain a profile of which genes are expressed in a given cell or tissue under defined conditions by means of cDNA arrays, which are thousands of unique DNA probes robotically deposited onto a solid matrix or "DNA chip". To profile gene expression in the tissue of interest, messenger RNA is isolated, copied into DNA labelled with a fluorescent dye and then used to probe the DNA chip to obtain an expression profile. A huge amount of data can be gathered in this manner, but to turn this into interpretable information requires considerable computing capacity—the processing and interpretation of data so obtained is known as bio-informatics. Profiling gene expression in various conditions may be useful diagnostically and may ultimately yield considerable information about the function of hitherto unidentified genes. Proteomics, the systematic study of all the proteins in a cell, tissue or organ, may ultimately be more useful than genomics. However, the technical hurdles are much greater, not least due to the vast number and complexity of the proteins to be studied. Improved methods for gel-separation of proteins and improved image analysis are likely to make study of the proteome a legitimate goal.

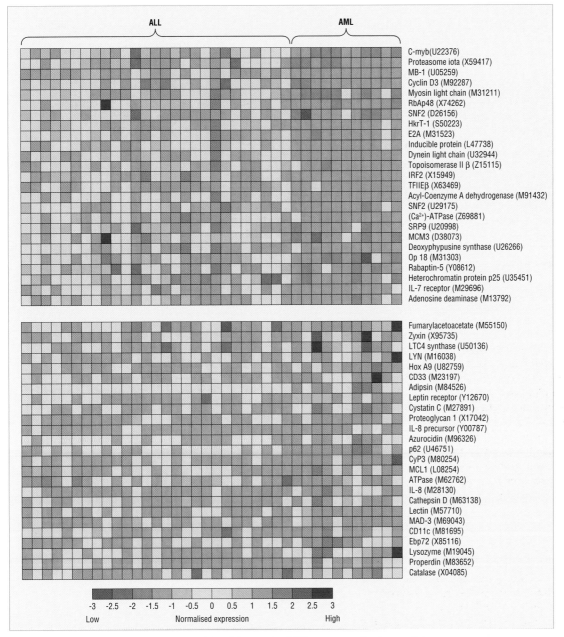

C-myb(U22376)
Proteasome iota (X59417)
MB-1 (U05259)
Cyclin D3 (M92287)
Myosin light chain (M31211)
RbAp48 (X74262)
SNF2 (D26156)
HkrT-1 (S50223)
E2A (M31523)
Inducible protein (L47738)
Dynein light chain (U32944)
Topoisomerase II β (Z15115)
IRF2 (X15949)
TFIIEβ (X63469)
Acyl-Coenzyme A dehydrogenase (M91432)
SNF2 (U29175)
(Ca²⁺)-ATPase (Z69881)
SRP9 (U20998)
MCM3 (D38073)
Deoxyphypusine synthase (U26266)
Op 18 (M31303)
Rabaptin-5 (Y08612)
Heterochromatin protein p25 (U35451)
IL-7 receptor (M29696)
Adenosine deaminase (M13792)

Fumarylacetoacetate (M55150)
Zyxin (X95735)
LTC4 synthase (U50136)
LYN (M16038)
Hox A9 (U82759)
CD33 (M23197)
Adipsin (M84526)
Leptin receptor (Y12670)
Cystatin C (M27891)
Proteoglycan 1 (X17042)
IL-8 precursor (Y00787)
Azurocidin (M96326)
p62 (U46751)
CyP3 (M80254)
MCL1 (L08254)
ATPase (M62762)
IL-8 (M28130)
Cathepsin D (M63138)
Lectin (M57710)
MAD-3 (M69043)
CD11c (M81695)
Ebp72 (X85116)
Lysozyme (M19045)
Properdin (M83652)
Catalase (X04085)

-3 -2.5 -2 -1.5 -1 -0.5 0 0.5 1 1.5 2 2.5 3
Low   Normalised expression   High

Figure 15.3 Microarray technology allows analysis of thousands of different genes simultaneously

Haemoglobinopathies

The identification of the precise mutations associated with many forms of hereditary anaemias will allow routine characterisation by nucleic acid sequence analysis, facilitating the use of disease specific diagnostic tests based on polymerase chain reaction. This will provide more precise prognostic information for affected individuals as well as accurate identification of affected embryos. As reliable prenatal diagnosis at an early stage will be available, so will an increasing range of prenatal treatment options.

For patients affected by hereditary anaemias such as sickle cell disease and thalassaemia, advances in transplantation immunology are likely to permit transplantation across tissue barriers with reduced immunosuppression, making bone marrow transplantation a treatment option for all affected patients. In addition, gene therapy for these disorders could provide another potentially curative strategy, although the genetic correction of hereditary anaemias still presents complex challenges. In sickle cell disease, for example, delivery of normal copies of the

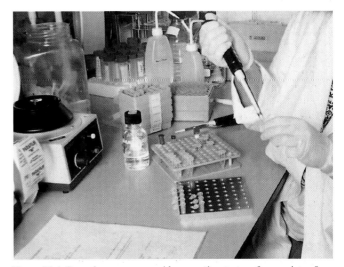

Figure 15.4 Gene therapy may provide a curative strategy for a variety of disorders, including haemoglobinopathies, coagulation disorders, and other single gene disorders

67

β globin gene to haemopoietic stem cells will be insufficient for cure. As continued Hb S production would be damaging, the mutated β globin genes must also be removed. Stem cell surgery techniques might be used to achieve such an aim.

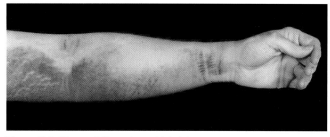

Figure 15.5 Haemophilic patient with inhibitors and severe spontaneous bleeding. Currently the development of inhibitors represents one of the biggest problems facing patients with haemophilia

Haemophilia

As specific mutations have now been identified to account for a large proportion of patients with haemophilia, routine characterisation of all haemophilias by direct sequence analysis is likely. This will facilitate accurate carrier diagnosis and thus the use of disease specific diagnostic tests based on polymerase chain reaction for accurate identification of affected embryos. As for the inherited anaemias, several prenatal treatments are likely to become available.

Dependence on blood products with the attendant risk of viral transmission has been disastrous for many patients with haemophilia, but this is unlikely to be a problem in the future. Recombinant human factor VIII is already available, recombinant coagulation factor VIIa is improving the prospects for haemophilic patients with inhibitors to factor VIII, and the development of other recombinant coagulation factors will ultimately obviate the need to use fractionated human blood. Definitive gene therapy of haemophilia also has excellent prospects. Haemophilia is known to be curable by liver transplantation, indicating that it should also be curable by genetic modification of host cells to produce normal factor VIII. Regulation of gene expression is not thought to be a critical issue as a moderate excess of factor VIII has no known procoagulant effect. Theoretically, production of only a small amount, perhaps 5%, of the required coagulation protein should be enough to convert clinically severe into clinically mild haemophilia. There are concerns that cells producing factor VIII might be recognised as "foreign" by the patient and rejected. The first clinical study of gene therapy for haemophilia A to be published, in which fibroblasts engineered to produce FVIII were implanted intraperitoneally, did not set out to provide an answer to this question.

There are also concerns relating to the generation of coagulation factor inhibitors, thus recruitment of patients to the early studies should proceed with great caution. A number of clinical studies of gene therapy in both haemophilia A and B are now ongoing, employing retrovirus, adenovirus and adeno-associated virus vectors.

Haematological malignancy

An understanding of the molecular mechanism of malignant transformation in malignant disorders forms the basis for improved diagnostic sensitivity and the monitoring of minimal residual disease and paves the way for more directed treatment

> **Box 15.2 Clinical trials of gene therapy in haemophilia**
>
> A number of phase I clinical trials of gene therapy for haemophilia A and B are ongoing or completed. They illustrate well the different gene delivery systems under investigation—the safest and most effective method of gene delivery remains to be determined
>
> - **Transkaryotic Therapy Inc.**
>   Six subjects received omental implantation of autologous fibroblasts modified ex vivo by transfection of DNA encoding B-domain deleted human FVIII
> - **Chiron**
>   A replication defective Moloney murine leukaemia virus vector delivering B-domain deleted human FVIII is being used
> - **Avigen**
>   Subjects with haemophilia B receive intramuscular injection of adeno-associated virus vector encoding human FIX
> - **Genstar**
>   This study is the first human trial to employ a "gutless" adenoviral vector. The vector will deliver full length human FVIII cDNA under the control of the highly liver-specific albumin promoter which should result in targeting of FVIII expression to the liver

(a)

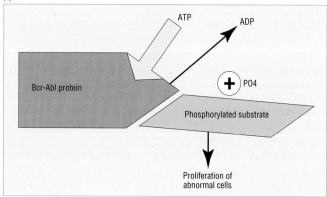

(b)

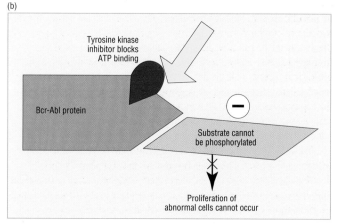

Figure 15.6 (a) Aberrant protein Bcr-Abl is produced in CML cells as a result of translocation of material from chromosome 9 to chromosome 22. It binds ATP then transfers phosphate groups to tyrosine residues on various substrate proteins. Downstream events lead to proliferation of the CML cells. (b) When STI571 binds to the ATP binding site of Bcr-Abl, the tyrosine kinase activity of this protein is inhibited and the events leading to proliferation of the CML cells cannot occur

Box 15.3 Success of anti-CD20 antibody therapy in lymphoma

Humanised antibody
- No anti-antibody immune reactions—permits multiple administrations

Multiple potential effector mechanisms
- Fixes complement
- Elicits ADCC reaction
- Binds to Fc receptors on effector cells

CD20 target restricted to B cells
- Transient depletion of normal B cells seen during therapy has minimal clinical consequences

Well tolerated
- Adverse reactions are mostly related to the infusion of the drug. Late adverse reactions are uncommon and have been mostly immune phenomena

Box 15.4 The future of antibody therapy for lymphoma?

Radioimmunotherapy
- The use of monoclonal antibodies to deliver radioisotopes to the target cells holds great promise and is poised to join "mainstream" therapies for lymphoma

Antibody delivery of immunotoxins
- Target antigens which are internalised are needed for this approach

Targeted delivery of oncolytic viruses via viral display of single chain antibodies
- In vitro studies and work in animal models suggest this may be a feasible approach

Novel target antigens
- Target antigens other than CD20 for which this approach is being developed clinically include CD22, HLA-DR, and CD52

Table 15.2 Scientific techniques and approaches that have made major contributions to modern haematology

Technique	Applications in haematology
Gene cloning and sequencing allow identification, characterisation, and manipulation of genes responsible for specific products or diseases	Elucidation of the molecular pathology of disease and diagnostic tests based on the polymerase chain reaction
Polymerase chain reaction is a highly sensitive and versatile technique for amplifying very small quantities of DNA. Amplification of RNA molecules is possible after initial reverse transcription of RNA into DNA (RT-PCR)	Rapid diagnosis of infectious diseases in immunocompromised patients (for example, hepatitis C); minimal residual disease detection in haematological malignancies where the molecular defect is known; carrier detection and antenatal diagnosis in haemophilias and hereditary anaemias
Monoclonal antibodies allow immunohistochemistry of tissue and cells, analysis and cell sorting with fluorescence activated cell sorter (FACS), and cell purification	Increased diagnostic precision, "positive purging," ex vivo gene delivery, and ex vivo expansion of progenitor cells are possible as a result of the fact that populations of haemopoietic cells containing a high proportion of primitive progenitors can be isolated
Mammalian tissue culture and gene transfer to mammalian cells provide methods for studying gene expression. Reporter genes can be used to study gene expression in cell lines in vitro. Transgenic animals can be created by inserting intact or manipulated genes into the germ line of an animal providing an in vivo model of gene function	Allows gene therapy, tissue engineering, and study of gene expression and function
Protein engineering and construction of recombinant proteins allow production of large quantities of human proteins. Proteins with modified or novel functions can be rationally designed and produced	Recombinant drugs (for example, the haemopoietic growth factors), antibody engineering to produce therapeutic antibodies, recombinant blood products free from risk of viral contamination

interventions, including the eventual possibility of targeting the causative genetic defects. The new genetic information available from genomic studies may eventually lead to new, genetic classifications of malignancies.

New pharmaceuticals based on our new understandings are already being developed the knowledge that deregulation of the tyrosine kinase activity of the Bcr-Abl fusion protein is the mechanism for oncogenesis in CML has led to the development of a new drug therapy, STI 571. This Abl-specific tyrosine kinase inhibitor has now demonstrated the potential of molecularly targeted therapies, and it is likely that the number of novel compounds will increase. The remarkable therapeutic success of monoclonal antibodies against the CD20 antigen in the treatment of lymphoma also paves the way for further therapeutic success with antibody therapies. More new biological agents will be developed that exploit the underlying mechanism of malignancy. A good example of this is the therapeutic use of replicative agents, such as oncolytic viruses, whose cytolytic capability is conditional upon some feature confined to malignant cells.

An increasing understanding of the role of the immune system in the elimination of haematological malignancies should also lead to more subtle approaches to therapy. It is clear that although current chemotherapy regimens do not eliminate all malignant cells, some patients can be cured after such conventional therapy and that a graft versus malignancy effect exists for most haematological malignancies. Strategies aimed at enhancing the immune response to malignant cells such as, for example, idiotypic vaccination in lymphoma, are likely to play an important role, particularly in the setting of minimal residual disease. An understanding that novel therapies must be developed in the context of existing treatment and that the right time to apply such therapies may not always be in the terminal stages of malignant disease is emerging.

Enhancement of the safety of existing effective treatments and increasing the number of people to whom they are applicable will remain an important aspect of progress in the treatment of haematological malignancy. We are likely to see

effective therapies applied to a increasing number of patients of advancing age and co-morbidity due to significant reductions in toxicity. Transplantation across HLA barriers has been demonstrated in a number of animal models. The use of non-myeloablative conditioning regimens should significantly reduce the toxicity of therapies which are known to be effective "Pharmacogenomics" may offer us the opportunity to identify the genetic mechanisms that affect the response to individual chemotherapy drugs in any given patient, so that those drugs or combinations of drugs offering the best therapeutic index for a particular person and their tumour can be used.

Box 15.5 Glossary

General molecular biology
- Recombinant DNA—Any DNA sequence that does not occur naturally but is formed by joining DNA segments from different sources
- Polymerase chain reaction—Process by which genes or gene segments can be rapidly, conveniently, and accurately copied, producing up to 10^{12} copies of the original sequence in a few hours
- Reverse transcription—Process by which RNA is used as a template for the production of a DNA copy
- Transcription factor—Protein that is able to bind to chromosomal DNA close to a gene and thereby regulates the expression of the gene

Haematology and immunology
- Stem cell—Pluripotent cell that has the ability to renew itself or differentiate. The haemopoietic stem cell gives rise to all lineages of haemopoietic cells
- Minimal residual disease—Cancer that is still present in the body after treatment but remains undetectable by conventional means—for example, light microscopy
- Immunophenotype—The cell surface markers on any given cell detected by the use of monoclonal antibodies
- Genomics—The systematic study of the human genome
- Proteomics—The systematic study of the human proteome
- Apoptosis—Programmed cell death
- Adoptive immunotherapy—The transfer of immune cells for therapeutic benefit
- Transgenic animals—Animals with an intact or manipulated gene inserted into their germline

Further reading
- Emilien G, Ponchon M, Caldas C, Isaacson O, Maloteaux JM. Impact of genomics on drug discovery and clinical medicine. *QJM* 2000;93(7):391-423.
- Ilidge TM, Bayne MC. Antibody therapy of lymphoma. *Expert Opin Pharmacother* 2001;2(6):953-61.
- Mannucci PM, Tuddenham EG. The hemophilias—from royal genes to gene therapy. *N Engl J Med* 2001;344(23):1773-9.
- Mauro MJ, O'Dwyer M, Heinrich MC, Druker BJ. STI571: a paradigm of new agents for cancer therapeutics. *J Clin Oncol* 2002;20(1):325-34.
- Miller DG, Stamatoyannopoulos G. Gene therapy for hemophilia. *N Engl J Med* 2001;344(23):1782-4.
- Roth DA, Tawa NE Jr, O'Brien JM, Treco DA, Selden RF. Nonviral transfer of the gene encoding coagulation factor VIII in patients with severe hemophilia A. *N Engl J Med* 2001;344(23):1735-42.
- Shipp MA, Ross KN, Tamayo P *et al*. Diffuse large B-cell lymphoma outcome prediction by gene-expression profiling and supervised machine learning. *Nat Med* 2002;8(1):68-74.

Figure 15.3 is reproduced from Aitman (*BMJ* 2001;323:611-15) and is adapted from Golub TR, Slonim DK, Tamayo P, Huard C, Gaasenbeek M, Mesirov JP, *et al*. Molecular classification of cancer: class discovery and class prediction by gene expression monitoring (*Science* 1999;286:531-7).

Index

page numbers in *italics* refer to tables and boxed text, those in **bold** refer to figures

Index

heparin 46
 disseminated intravascular coagulation 63
 low molecular weight 46
 unfractionated 46
heparin-induced thrombocytopenia 30, 32
heparinoids, synthetic 32
hereditary spherocytosis 13
herpes simplex virus 55
herpes zoster virus 55
 chronic lymphocytic leukaemia 64
HLA barriers 70
HLA matching 52
 developments 56
Hodgkin's disease 47, 50
homocysteine 6
 assay 7
HPA-1 29, 59
human genome sequence 65
human parvovirus B19 57
human platelet antigen 1a (HPA1a) 29, 59
hydrops 57
hydroxo-cobalamin 8
hydroxyurea 7, 10, 15, 16
 chronic myeloid leukaemia 21
 myelodysplastic syndromes 36
hyperviscosity syndrome 61
hypochromic anaemia 2
hypoparathyroidism 5

idiopathic thrombocytopenic purpura 29
 adults 32
 childhood 31–2
ileal resection 5
imatinib mesylate 19, 21, 22
immunoglobulins 63
 heavy chains 42
 multiple myeloma 37, 39
immunological impairment 63–4
immunophenotype 70
immunotherapy, adoptive 70
infants
 anaemia associated with infection 57
 β thalassaemia 57–8
 haematological disorders 57–9
 haemoglobinopathies 57–8
 haemostasis disorders 58
 sickle cell disease 58
 thrombocytopenia 58–9
infection
 anaemia 60
 asplenic patients 64
 chronic lymphocytic leukaemia 64
 fetal 57
 immunological impairment 63–4
 infant 58
 maternal 57
 sickle cell crisis 62
infertility 6
interferon α 15, 16, 21
interleukin 1β (IL-1β) 37
interleukin 6 (IL-6) 37
intestinal stagnant loop syndrome 5
intravenous immunoglobulin 32, 58, 59
 chronic lymphocytic leukaemia 64
intrinsic factor 5
 antibodies 7
iron deficiency 1–2
iron deficiency anaemia 1–4
 diagnosis 2
 elderly people 59
 laboratory investigations 2
 management 3

iron metabolism 1
iron replacement therapy 3–4
iron sorbitol injection 3
iron supplements
 elderly people 59
 prophylactic 4

kernicterus 57

leucocytosis 35
leucoerythroblastic blood picture 16–17
leukaemia 16
 acute 23–7
  chemotherapy 25–6
  classification 23–4
  hyperviscosity syndrome 61
  incidence 24
  investigations 24–5
  management 25–7
  multi-drug resistant genotype 27
  presentation 24
  survival 26
  toxicity of therapy 27
 acute promyelocytic 63
 adult T cell 26
 plasma cell 42
 predisposition syndromes 28
 see also acute lymphoblastic leukaemia; Burkitt's
  lymphoma/leukaemia; chronic lymphocytic
  leukaemia; chronic myeloid leukaemia;
  chronic myelomonocytic leukaemia
leukapheresis 61
liver disease 44–5
liver transplantation 68
lupus anticoagulant 46
lymphocytes, donor infusion 56
lymphoma 41
 B cell 49, 50
 CD20 antigen monoclonal antibodies 69
 cord compression 62
 extranodal 48
 follicular 47–8
 idiotypic vaccination 69
 karyotyping 50
 lymphoblastic 49
 malignant 47–50
 marginal zone 48
 staging 47
 T cell 49
lymphoproliferative disorders 45

macrocytic anaemia 5–8
macrocytosis 5, 6
 benign familial 7
macroglobulinaemia 41
malabsorption 2
 folate 6
 vitamin B12 5
 vitamin K 45
malaria 57
malignancy 3
 anaemia 60
 disseminated 45
 elderly people 60
 gastrointestinal 59
 haematological 68–70
 regression 48
maltoma 48
May Hegglin anomaly **28,** 29
megakaryocytes 20, 28
megaloblastic anaemia 5, 6
 elderly people 59–60

Index